OVERWEIGHT,
OBESITY AND HEALTH

OVERWEIGHT, OBESITY AND HEALTH

Web Resource Guide for Consumers, Healthcare Providers, Patients, and Physicians

Eugene A. DeFelice, M.D., F.A.P.M.

Writers Club Press

New York Lincoln Shanghai

Overweight, Obesity and Health
Web Resource Guide for Consumers, Healthcare Providers, Patients,
and Physicians

Writers Club Press
an imprint of iUniverse, Inc.

For information address:
iUniverse
2021 Pine Lake Road, Suite 100
Lincoln, NE 68512
www.iuniverse.com

ISBN: 0-595-26240-6

Printed in the United States of America

Dedication

This book is dedicated to two people instrumental in its publication.

Ms. Maryanne Harvey, M.S., Section Chief, New York State Department of Health.

Maryanne, my friend, has devoted most of her professional life to the betterment of the health and welfare of others as a leader in the New York State Department of Health for many years.

Without her friendship, encouragement, inspiration, dedication, able professional assistance, and expertise in preparing, editing, and submission of the manuscript, publication of this book would not have been possible.

Mr. Benjamin DeFelice, Literary Agent

Ben, my brother, world traveler, racanteur extraordinarie, friend and helping hand to many throughout his life, acted as my Literary Agent regarding the publication of this book. He enlisted in the Maritime Service in World War II, answering the call of duty early in the hostilities, volunteering repeatedly for a number of dangerous missions without regard for his own life. Thus, he is regarded by all those who know him well as a "true patriot" and a "man for all seasons".

As two individuals who have done so much for so many, their life examples have inspired me to write this book in the hope that it also will prove helpful to others, enabling them to live a healthier, happier and longer life.

Contents

Acknowledgements

The Author acknowledges that the Web resources listed in chapter 9, and additional ones cited in the text, provided the bulk of information on overweight, obesity and health-related complications used in this book.

Preface

Most individuals do not pay sufficient attention to their health. Rather they usually tend to:

> Squander health in search of wealth
> They work and toil and save
> Then squander wealth in search of health
> But find an early grave.

> Anonymous

To prevent overweight, obesity, and health-related complications, or to overcome them once they have occurred, one needs to become concerned, informed, knowledgeable, and:

> Take charge, control and responsibility for their health
> Obtain reliable information about overweight and obesity
> Follow steps to prevent occurrence whenever possible
> Seek professional intervention if prevention fails, and
> Employ effective management as soon as possible.

> Eugene A. DeFelice, MD

First, one needs to ask the right questions, and obtain current, comprehensive, reliable, and useful information in order to become informed and knowledgeable. In this regard, it has been said:

> I keep six honest serving men
> They taught me all I knew
> Their names are What and Why and When
> And How and Where and Who
>
> Rudyard Kipling

Next, an intelligent person should want to know all there is to know about overweight, obesity, and health-related complications, and profit accordingly. To do otherwise is just not in one's best interests. A great physician once said:

> I have always believed that intelligent people—
> not only wish to know as much as possible
> about any ailment they may have—but also that
> such people are entitled to know everything
> that is known about such ailments.
>
> George Crile, MD

The Internet/Web provides key resources by which to easily obtain available information on overweight, obesity and health-related complications. Numerous Web resources exist from which to obtain almost all, if not all, the information and expert opinion that one may need to become informed.

In fact, it is now widely recognized that:

> Healthcare is not what it use to be
> Healthcare is not even what it ought to be
> Healthcare on the web has grown to be
> Healthcare available for all as it should be.

Eugene A. DeFelice, MD

This book provides a very useful guide by which one can quickly and easily search the Web and obtain current, comprehensive, reliable and useful information on overweight, obesity and health-related complications. With such information, one can take charge, control and responsibility for their own health, and make informed decisions with their physician/healthcare provider, and live a healthier, happier, longer and more enjoyable and productive life.

Chapter I addresses: Overweight/Obesity: The Epidemic. Chapter II covers: Classification/Methods Used. Chapter 3 discusses: Causes/Pathogenesis. Chapter 4 outlines: Prevention and Methods used. Chapter 5 explains: Health Risks/Complications. Chapter 6 involves: Diagnosis. Chapter 7 provides information on: Treatment. Chapter 8 concerns useful ways of: Searching the Web. Chapter 9 presents the: Author's List: Key Web Resources. Chapter 10 highlights Web resources for: Dictionary, Medical Encyclopedia and Glossary of Terms.

There is no one best answer for any question regarding overweight/obesity and health-related complications. One must ultimately obtain the best information available from a variety of sources and decide what is "right/best" under their particular circumstances of the moment in conjunction/consultation with their physician/healthcare provider.

It is estimated that well over 200 million people now consult the Web for healthcare information and the vast majority regard such as useful. I trust you will, too.

Eugene A. DeFelice, MD

1. Overweight/Obesity: The Epidemic

1.1 Definition

The American Association of Clinical Endocrinology (AACE) and American College of Endocrinology (ACE) regard obesity as a complex, multifactorial chronic disease characterized by an excess of body fat that requires long-term, continued treatment, support, and follow-up. Men with more then 25% and women with more than 35% body fat, are considered to be obese. Those with a body mass index 25.0-29.9 are considered overweight and 30 or greater as obese. Obesity not only has a number of causes, most likely representing different disorders combined under one label, but also may cause other serious complications/diseases as well.

One may have a body weight within the desired norm for height and frame size and still have a high percentage of undesirable fat in the body. In addition, body weight for a given height can exceed the norm for certain individuals because of large muscle mass (e.g., in weight lifters, athletes, etc.) and such persons are not considered to be clinically obese and complications may not be readily discernable. Therefore, a physician should be consulted to determine the presence or absence of obesity and complications.

Healthy weight ranges, issued by the Dietary Guidelines Advisory Committee of the US Department of Agriculture Food and Nutrition Information Center, are considered to be useful and widely accepted body weight standards for adults. They are available at: http://www.usda.gov/fnic.

For further information, consult the report on *Understanding Adult Obesity* by the National Institute of Diabetes, Digestive and Kidney Diseases (NIDDK) at: http://www.niddk.nih.gov/health/nutrit/pubs/unders.htm.

1.2   Facts/Statistics

1.2.1 Adults

The US Surgeon General's Office/U.S. Government state that:
- 61% of adults in the United States are overweight/obese, an epidemic of epic proportions
- over 300,000 deaths each year in the US are associated with obesity
- heart disease, certain types of cancer, type 2 diabetes mellitus (non insulin- dependent), stroke, arthritis, breathing problems, and psychological disorders such as depression, etc., are recognized complications of obesity
- increases in overweight and obesity cut across all ages, racial and ethnic groups, and both genders
- economic costs, direct and indirect, for obesity in the US are in the billions
- the prevalence of overweight and obesity increases until about age 60, after which it begins to decline
- in women, overweight and obesity are higher among members of racial and ethnic minority populations than in non-Hispanic white women
- in men, Mexican Americans have a higher prevalence of overweight and obesity than non-Hispanic whites or non-Hispanic blacks
- 69% of non-Hispanic black women are overweight or obese compared to 58% of non-Hispanic black men
- 62% of non-Hispanic white men are overweight or obese compared with 47% of non-Hispanic white women
- for all racial and ethnic groups combined, women of lower socioeconomic status (income <130% of poverty threshold) are approximately 50% more likely to be overweight or obese compared to those of higher socioeconomic status

- less than 1/3 of adults engage in the recommended amounts of physical activity—most living sedentary lives. In fact 40% of adults in the US do not participate in any leisure time physical activity
- overweight and obesity primarily result from an imbalance involving excessive calorie consumption and/or inadequate physical activity
- for each individual, body weight usually is the result of a combination of genetic, metabolic, behavioral, environmental, cultural and socioeconomic influences
- behavioral and environmental factors are large contributors to overweight and obesity and provide the greatest opportunity for actions and interventions designed for prevention and treatment
- adults should accumulate at least 30 minutes of physical activity most days (4-5) of the week. More may be needed to prevent weight gain, to lose weight or to maintain weight loss. Physical activity is very important in preventing and treating overweight and obesity and is extremely helpful in producing and maintaining weight loss, especially when combined with healthy eating and behavior modification

An October 2002 report from the Centers for Disease Control and Prevention (http://www.cdc.gov) indicates that two thirds of adults (65%) are now considered to be overweight and one third are regarded as medically obese (circa 59 million adults). In addition, around 5% of adults are believed to be severely obese (e.g., BMI over 40).

For additional information consult:

Surgeon General's Office
- Report on: *Call to Action to Prevent and Decrease Overweight and Obesity* http://www.surgeongeneral.gov/topics/obesity/default.htm

- Report on: *Overweight and Obesity: At a Glance*
  http://www.surgeongeneral.gov/topics/obesity/calltoaction/
  fact_glance.htm
- Report on: *Overweight and Obesity: Health Consequences*
  http://www.surgeongeneral.gov/topics/obesity/calltoaction/
  fact_ consequences.htm
- Report on: *Overweight and Obesity: A Vision for the Future*
  http://www.surgeongeneral.gov/topics/obesity/calltoaction/
  fact_vision.htm
- Report on: *Surgeon General's Healthy Weight Advice for Consumers*
  http://www.surgeongeneral.gov/topics/obesity/calltoaction/
  fact_advice.htm

National Center for Chronic Disease Prevention and Health Promotion
- Report on: *Frequently Asked Questions (And Answers)*
  http://www.cdc.gov/nccdphp/dnpa/obesity/faq.htm

National Heart, Lung and Blood Institute
- Report on: *Clinical Guidelines on the Identification, Evaluation, and Treatment of Overweight and Obesity in Adults—Executive Summary*
  http://www.nhlbi.nih.gov/guidelines/obesity/sum_evid.htm

1.2.2. Children and Adolescents

The Surgeon General's Office states that:
- over 13% of children aged 6-11 years and 14% of adolescents aged 12-19 years are overweight or obese in the United States. This prevalence has nearly tripled for adolescents in the past 2 decades.
- overweight adolescents have a 70% chance of becoming overweight or obese adults. This increases to 80% if one or more parent is overweight or obese.
- risk factors for heart disease, such as high cholesterol and high blood pressure, are reported to occur with increased frequency in

overweight and obese children and adolescents compared to those with a healthy weight.
- type 2 diabetes mellitus, previously considered an adult onset disease, has increased dramatically in overweight and obese children and adolescents.
- the more immediate consequence of overweight or obesity as perceived by children and adolescents themselves is social discrimination. This is often associated with poor self-esteem and depression.

Causes of Overweight and Obesity in Children and Adolescents include:
- generally caused by lack of physical activity, unhealthy eating patterns, or a combination of the two, with genetics and lifestyle also playing important roles in determining weight.
- television, the computer, and video game time contribute to inactive lifestyle.
- 43% of adolescents watch more than 2 hours of television each day.
- children/ adolescents have become sedentary and less active as they grow older.

Determination of Overweight and Obesity in Children and Adolescents includes:
- doctors and other health professionals are in the best position to determine whether a child's or adolescent's weight is healthy. They can help rule out rare medical problems as the cause.
- health professionals often use a BMI "growth chart" to help assess overweight and obesity in children and adolescent.

General Suggestions include:
- let your child know he or she is loved and appreciated whatever his or her weight. An overweight or obese child knows better than anyone

else that he or she has a weight problem. Overweight children need support, acceptance, and encouragement from their parents.

- focus on your child's health and positive qualities, not your child's weight
- try not to make your child feel different if he or she is overweight or obese, and focus on gradually changing your family's physical activities and eating habits
- be a good role model for your child. If your child sees you enjoying healthy foods and physical activity, he or she is more likely to do the same now and for the rest of his or her life.
- realize that an appropriate goal for many overweight or obese children is to maintain their current weight while growing normally in height.

Physical Activity Suggestions include:
- be physically active. It is recommended that Americans accumulate at least 30-60 minutes—children 60 minutes—of moderate physical activity/exercise most days of the week. Even greater amounts of physical activity/exercise may be necessary for the prevention of weight gain, for weight loss, or for sustaining weight loss.
- plan family activities that provide everyone with exercise and enjoyment.
- provide a safe environment for your children and their friends to play actively.
- encourage physical exercise, swimming, biking, skating, ball sports, and other fun physical activities.
- reduce the amount of time you and your family spend in sedentary activities such as watching TV or playing video games, cards, etc. Limit TV time to around 1 hour a day.

Healthy Eating Suggestions include:
- follow *Dietary Guidelines for Healthy Eating*
  http://www.health.gov/dietaryguidelines
- guide your family's choices rather than dictate foods
- encourage your child to eat only when hungry and to eat slowly
- eat meals together as often as possible
- cut down on the amount of fat and calories in your family's/child's diet
- don't place your child on a restrictive diet
- avoid the use of food as a reward
- avoid withholding food as punishment
- children should be encouraged to drink water and to limit intake of beverages with added sugars such as soft drinks, fruit juice drinks and sports drinks
- plan for only healthy snacks
- stock the refrigerator with fat-free or low-fat milk, fresh fruit, and vegetables instead of soft drinks or snacks that are high in fat, calories, or added sugars, and low in essential nutrients
- aim to eat at least 5 servings of fruit and vegetables each day
- discourage eating meals or snacks while watching TV
- eating a healthy breakfast is a good way to start the day and may prove to be important in achieving and maintaining a healthy weight

If Your Child is Overweight or Obese, consider:
- many overweight children and some mildly obese, who are still growing, will not need to lose weight but can reduce their rate of weight gain so they can "grow into" their normal weight.
- your child's diet should be safe and nutritious. It should include all of the Recommended Dietary Allowances (RDAs) for vitamins,

minerals, and protein, carbohydrates, and fats, and contain foods from the major Food Guide Pyramid groups. Any weight-loss diet for an obese child should be low in calories only, not in essential nutrients.

- even with extremely overweight/obese children, weight loss should be gradual.
- crash diets and diet pills can compromise growth and are not recommended
- weight loss during a diet is frequent regained unless children are motivated to change their eating habits and physical activity levels for a lifetime.
- weight control must be considered a lifelong effort.
- any weight management program for children should be supervised by a physician.

For additional information, consult the Surgeon General's Office report on: *Overweight in Children and Adolescents* at:
http://www.surgeongenreal.gov/topics/obesity/calltoaction/
fact_adolescents.htm

Further discussion of overweight/obesity in children and adolescents is beyond the scope of this book. For additional information it is recommended that the reader consult a pediatric or family physician who is knowledgeable and experienced in the field.

2. Classification/Methods Used

2.1 Introduction

The degree of overweight, obesity and body fat content are estimated clinically by measuring body mass index (BMI), waist and hip circumferences and their ratio, and skin-fold thickness in selected areas.

All of the methods together provide a reasonably good estimate of over-weight, obesity, and body fat content and distribution as indicated in Table I below:

Table I Comparison of BMI, Waist/Hip Ratio, and Skin-fold Thickness

	BMI	Waist/Hip Ratio	Skin-fold Thickness
Cost	Low	Low	Low
Use	Easy	Easy	Easy
Accuracy	High	Moderate	Moderate
Fat location	No	Yes	Yes

Each method alone has its limitations. Together, they provide information that is clinically useful not only in classification and diagnosis, but also in following and documenting the course of treatment.

A number of other methods of estimating body fat and distribution are available but these are more costly and difficult to use and thus employed primarily in research centers. See Wang, Z.M., et al. Am. J. Clin. Nutr. 61:457-465, 1995 for a discussion of these methods.

For additional information regarding classification of overweight and obesity, consult:

National Center for Chronic Disease Prevention and Health Promotion
* Report on: *Overweight and Obesity*
  http://www.cdc.gov/nccdphp/dnpa/obesity/basics.htm
* Report on: *Body Mass Index* (BMI)
  http://www.cdc.gov/nccdphp/dnpa/obesity/bmi.htm

National Heart, Lung and Blood Institute
- Report on: *Body Mass Index Table*
  http://www.nhlbi.nih.gov/guidelines/obesity/bmi_tbl2.htm
- Report on: *Body Mass Index-for-Age (Children)*
  http://www.cdc.gov/nccdphp/dnpa/bmi/bmi–for–age.htm
- Report on: *Classification of Overweight and Obesity by BMI, Waist Circumference and Associated Disease Risks*
  http://www.nhlbi.nih.gov/health/public/heart/obesity/lose_wt/bmi_dis.htm

2.2   Body Mass Index

An expert panel, convened by the National Institute of Health in 1998 recommended that Body Mass Index (BMI) be used to classify overweight and obesity. This was done because the BMI:

1. correlates well with total body fat for the majority of people
2. correlates with the risk of disease complications and death. For example, heart disease increases with increasing BMI in all population groups
3. calculation is simple, rapid, and inexpensive with a hand or Web resource calculator, or using a table/nomogram

The BMI is a measure of weight in relation to height determined by the following formulas:

> BMI=weight in kilograms divided by height in meters squared, or
> BMI=weight in pounds divided by height in inches squared times 703

Tables are commonly used for estimating BMI such as the one provided by the National Heart, Lung, and Blood Institute at:
http://www.nhlbi.nih.gov/guidelines/obesity/bmi_tbl.htm

For a "Body Mass Index Calculator", consult:
CDC National Center for Chronic Disease Prevention and Health Promotion at:
http://www.cdc.gov/nccdphp/dnpa/bmi/calc-bmi.htm

CaloriesPerHour.com
http://www.caloriesperhour.com

Classification of overweight and obesity via the BMI generally is determined in adults as indicated in Table II below.

Table II Classification of Overweight/Obesity, and Medical Risk*

Classification	BMI	Medical Risk
• Healthy Weight	BMI 18.5-24.9	Very low risk
• Overweight	BMI 25.0-29.9	Low risk
• Obesity		
• Mild, Class I	BMI 30.0-34.9	Moderate risk
• Moderate, Class II	BMI 35.0-39.9	High risk
• Severe, Class III	BMI > 40.0	Very high risk

* for complications

In children and adolescents 6 to 19 years of age, overweight is defined as a sex-and-age-specific BMI at or above the 95th percentile, based on revised Centers for Disease Control and Prevention growth charts available at: http://www.cdc.gov/growthcharts

It should be recognized that the BMI has certain limitations. It can overestimate body fat in persons who are very muscular, and underestimate body fat in persons who have lost muscle mass such as the elderly. Therefore, a diagnosis of overweight or obesity needs to be made by a health professional experienced in the field.

2.3 Waist Circumference and Waist/Hip Ratio

Two basic fat distribution patterns exist in overweight and obese individuals. One is called android (apple-shaped or central, chiefly around the abdomen). The other is designated gynoid (pear-shaped or gluteofemoral, principally around the hips, buttocks, and thighs). These two types can be differentiated visually or classified by the waist-to-hip circumferences and ratio.

Waist circumference is a common measure used to assess abdominal fat content. The presence of excess body fat around the abdomen, when out of proportion to total body fat, is considered an independent predictor of risk of health complications.

For waist circumference, a tape measure is used to comfortably measure the distance around the smallest area of the abdomen below the rib cage and above the umbilicus (belly button). A waist circumference over 40 inches (102 centimeters) in men and 35 inches (88 centimeters) in women is considered to be android or central obesity, and is more closely correlated with significant health complications and premature death.

Hip circumference likewise also is measured with a tape measure. It is the distance comfortably measured around the body's hip area at the largest extension of the buttocks. Hip circumference greater than waist is designated gynoid or guteofemoral obesity.

Waist-to-hip ratio (WHR) is calculated as the waist divided by the hip circumference. For most people, carrying extra weight around their "middle" increases health risks, complications, and premature death more then carrying the extra weight around their hips, buttocks or thighs. However, overall obesity (increase in total body fat) is a greater risk for health complications than fat storage locations or waist-to-hip ratio.

For both men and women, a waist-to-hip ratio of 1.0 or higher is considered "at risk" or in the danger zone for health complications and premature death.

Waist-to-hip ratios of less than 0.8 in women and less than 1.0 in men are considered normal.

Note that for a person with a short stature (under 5 feet in height and a BMI of 35 or above), waist circumference standards for the general population may not apply.

For additional information on "Waist-to-Hip Calculator", consult: http://www.global-fitness.com/whrcalc_intro.html

2.4   Body Fat Skin Caliper

Fat accumulates extensively under the skin in overweight and obese individuals. Therefore, a useful and practical way to measure body fat percentage and distribution is by determining skin-fold thickness using a body fat skin caliper—a technique based on the time-honored "pinch an inch" method. Measuring skin-fold thickness in this manner is reported to compare reasonably well with the so-called "gold standard" method of underwater weighing—although there is disagreement on this point. The site usually chosen for skin-fold thickness measurement is the area approximately one inch above the right hip bone. At least three consecutive measurements usually are made at the chosen site and results averaged and compared to a standard chart to obtain an estimate of the percentage of body fat.

A rough clinical estimate of skin-fold thickness may be obtained by pinching the skin between the index finger and thumb, maintaining the gap formed between the two fingers as the hand is drawn away, and estimating the gap size with a ruler. A gap of over one-inch indicates excess fat, and the wider the gap over one inch, the greater the degree of body fat.

The Accumeasurefitness.com battery operated Fat Track Digital Skin-fold Caliper uses a patented floating code skin thickness measuring system for accuracy and repeatability of skin-fold thickness measurements in the hip, upper midsection and lower body areas for direct digital readouts of percent body fat. With this device, there is a digital "read out" and no more tables or charts to interpret.

For additional information and illustrations consult: http://www.accumeasurefitness.com.

3. Causes/Pathogenesis

3.1 Introduction

Individuals expend energy through basal or resting metabolism, thermal effects of meals, and physical activity/exercise. When more calories are consumed than expended, overweight and/or obesity result. However, the exact cause(s) of this imbalance is not well understood at this time. Nevertheless, some factors that may be regarded as causative for overweight and obesity may include: genetic, hormonal, environmental, and psychological factors.

3.2 Genetic Factors

Only a few very rare obesity disorders are considered to be primarily genetic in origin at this time. Examples include: Prader-Willi's and Carpenter's Syndromes, etc. as well as Lipodystrophy. Discussion of these rare types of overweight/obesity is beyond the scope of this book. Further information on these disorders may be obtained from the Office of Rare Diseases, National Institutes of Health at: http://www.rarediseases.info.nih.gov.

Several types of evidence available at this time indicate that, except in such rare cases cited above, genetic factors alone do not explain the epidemic of overweight and obesity now gripping the United States and the rest of the Western World. In fact, genetic factors are believed to account for only around 30% of weight. Whatever the genetic influence on overweight and obesity, such appears to be largely overshadowed by non-genetic factors in the vast majority of cases. Nevertheless it still needs to be recognized that some individuals are more susceptible to either weight gain or loss than others, and this cannot always be attributed to lack of adherence to dietary or physical activity regimens.

3.3 Hormonal Factors

3.3.1 Overview

Scientists suspect that human beings may have a number of genes and associated hormones that regulate the energy balance equation—the calories we consume versus the calories we burn through basal metabolism, thermogenesis, and physical activity. However, the role(s) hormones and genes play in overweight and obesity remains to be clarified.

Some hormonal causes of overweight and obesity have been recognized for many years. However, they are not common causes of overweight and obesity, and include such things as:

- Hypothyroidism—a deficiency of thyroid hormone(s) due to more than one cause.
- Cushing's Syndrome—an excess of adrenocortical hormone arising from internal or external causes.
- Polycystic Ovary Syndrome (Stein-Leventhal Syndrome)—due to complex hormonal effects

Polycystic ovary syndrome (PCOS), formerly known as the Stein-Leventhal Syndrome, was first described by two American gynecologists, Stein and Leventhal, in 1905. It is reported to affect up to 10% of women. It can start in adolescence or any time in a woman's reproductive life.

PCOS is a metabolic disorder in which abnormal hormone levels result in a number of problems including obesity, diabetes, heart disease, acne, excessive facial and body hair, uterine cancer, and infertility. In fact, PCOS appears to account for more than 50% of cases of female infertility. And over 50% of cases of PCOS become obese and have difficulty losing weight.

Two pituitary hormones, FSH and LH appear to be principally involved. Also, many women with PCOS have high blood levels of insulin, insulin resistance, and are prone to develop type 2 diabetes mellitus. And those with high blood levels of insulin and insulin resistance often gain weight even on a normal diet.

Blood levels of testosterone also are likely to be elevated, resulting in disturbing acne, hirsutism of the face, abdomen and chest, and male-pattern baldness that are difficult to treat successfully.

High levels of triglycerides and low levels of high density lipoprotein cholesterol plus high blood levels of insulin and insulin resistance found in many cases all increase the risk of heart disease and stroke.

Treatment is difficult and complicated at best. Some women with PCOS appear to be helped by birth control pills. Treatment of insulin resistance with diet, exercise, weight loss, and drugs may help to prevent diabetes and cardiovascular complications. Metformin appears to help restore hormonal balance, normal menstrual cycles, and improve insulin resistance, reducing steroid abnormalities in both the adrenals and ovaries. Depression, anxiety and stress are not uncommon PCOS complications requiring treatment.

Hypothyroidism, Cushing's Syndrome, and Polycystic Ovary Syndrome need to be ruled in, or out, in the diagnosis of overweight and obesity by appropriate laboratory tests and clinical examination, and managed accordingly. As they constitute special cases, they are beyond the scope of this book and will not be considered further.

For further information on hypothyroidism and Cushing's disease and PCOS, consult: Medlineplus, or the National Institutes of Health Web resources. Additional information on PCOS may be found at: http://www.pcosupport.org or http://www.webmd.com.

3.3.2 Insulin

Insulin, the so-called "master hormone" is secreted by the beta cells of the pancreas. It regulates the amount of glucose (sugar) in the blood and tissues, and determines how much fat may be stored in the body. Insulin resistance frequently accompanies overweight and obesity and must be effectively countered by diet, exercise, and certain drugs especially in patients with type 2 diabetes mellitus.

Aside from insulin that regulates sugar and fat metabolism/storage, the rest of the hormonal puzzle regarding the energy balancing act remains rudimentary and speculative at best at this time.

3.3.3 Leptin

Leptin derives its name from the Greek "leptos" meaning thin. Manufactured in fat cells of the body, leptin secretion sends satiety (fullness) signals to the hypothalamus—the brain's eating control center—to tell us to stop eating.

As one increases body fat deposition, fat cells "pump out" more leptin indicating that it is time to increase energy output and decrease caloric intake. In individuals who gain weight, a significant resistance to leptin's action(s) on the hypothalamus appears to occur. Also, when an overweight/obese individual loses weight and leptin levels decrease, the hypothalamus may misread this drop in leptin levels as a "starvation signal" causing increased eating and a regain of weight to occur.

Very rarely, individuals may have a genetic defect (in the so-called ob gene in fat tissue) whereby they are leptin deficient. Genetically leptin deficient individuals are reported to have a voracious appetite, do not feel full after a meal and develop obesity. Injections of leptin reduce their appetite and produce significant weight loss (around 50% of overweight in one year). In addition, leptin injections appear to stimulate physical activity in these individuals.

In contrast, obese individuals without this genetic leptin defect, have on average four times higher serum leptin levels compared to non obese persons. When such obese persons lose 10% of their initial body weight, serum leptin levels decrease by 55% on average. Also, when serum leptin levels are evaluated before and after meals, leptin concentrations do not change significantly in overweight and obese individuals.

Nevertheless, some clinical studies have shown that higher doses of leptin may produce some weight loss in obese patients.

Thus, the role of leptin in overweight and obesity needs further clarification. While leptin appears to show some promise for treating obese individuals with a genetic deficiency of leptin, it does not appear to be the "magic bullet" hoped for in the treatment of the vast majority of cases of overweight and obesity.

For additional information on leptin, the reader may consult:

Rockefeller University
• Report on: *Leptin Helps Body Regulate Fat, Links to Diet*
  http://www.rockefeller.edu/pubinfo/leptinlevel.nr.html

Weight.com
• Report on: *Leptin—Can Obese Mice Lead to Lean People*
  http://www.weight.com/Leptin.html

National Library of Medicine
• Search "Leptin"
  http://www.nlm.nih.gov

3.3.4 Ghrelin

Cells in the lining of the stomach release a hormone called ghrelin that causes an individual to feel hungry when the stomach is empty. Researchers report that human volunteers injected with ghrelin become ravenous and increase their food intake accordingly. Leptin appears to inform the body when to stop eating once sufficient fat is stored whereas ghrelin stimulates an individual to eat and store more fat.

When an individual diets and loses weight, ghrelin release induces feelings of hunger making the body feel it is starving and thus appears to encourage one to regain the weight lost. In weight loss studies with obese individuals, ghrelin was found to rise sharply in blood before meals and fall shortly after meals, further indicating that grehlin levels trigger the desire to eat. However, after a significant loss of body weight, ghrelin blood levels appear to rise leading one to regain weight lost and even more.

With gastric bypass surgical treatment of obesity, ghrelin blood levels are reported to be 77% lower than in normal-weight controls, and 72% lower than matched obese controls. Thus patients losing weight after gastric bypass surgery appear to have very low ghrelin blood levels compared to those who had lost the same amount of weight in non-surgical weight loss programs and those of normal weight. Also, ghrelin blood levels do not rise before meals in the gastric bypass surgical patients as in obese non-surgically treated patients.

Weight reduction brought about by caloric restriction causes ghrelin levels to increase. This suggests that ghrelin may contribute to the need to eat which makes long term success with dieting less likely.

The ghrelin story apparently has stirred efforts to find new agents that suppress the production of ghrelin, or block its stimulating effects on eating, and determine their efficacy and safety in the treatment of overweight and obesity. Such developments, however, will take a number of years to accomplish.

For additional information search "ghrelin" at:
http://www.ncbi.nlm.nih.gov/pubmed

3.3.5 PYY 3-36

PYY 3-36, the so-called satiety hormone, is reported to be released naturally by the cells in the digestive tract after every meal. Release of this hormone signals the feeding center/circuits in the hypothalamus, conveying a sense of satiety (fullness) that reduces the urge to eat.

Volunteers receiving intravenous injections of PYY 3-36 are reported to consume, on average, about one third fewer calories in the following 24-hour period. Also, they reported a 40% drop in perceived levels of hunger in the 12 hour period after receiving the drug.

While this hormone was first extracted from pig's gut in Stockholm, Sweden in 1983, it is only very recently that PYY 3-36 was found to suppress appetite in humans. Some feel it may represent a major step forward on the road to the development of a new effective treatment for overweight and obesity.

Further studies are needed to determine if PYY 3-36 is effective subcutaneously, and whether certain foods may preferentially cause its release and limit appetite.

For additional information, consult PubMed at: http://www.ncbi.nlm.nih.gov/pubmed (and search "PYY 3-36").

While there may be certain inferences from the research to date regarding these hormonal factors and others that may be involved in overweight and obesity, any new drugs that may flow from this information are regarded as still many years away from the marketplace. In the meantime, experts seem to agree that the safest approach to overweight and obesity centers around eating less and exercising more until further research dictates otherwise.

3.4   Environmental Factors

Social factors, unhealthy lifestyle, lack of physical activity, and psychological influences are believed to play a significant role in the development of overweight and obesity.

People of low socioeconomic status tend to suffer from overweight and obesity more often. Certain cultural and ethnic factors also appear to have a significant influence. Latinos, African-Americans and Native Americans have been found to be more prone to develop overweight and obesity.

Consuming an unhealthy diet and high dietary fat intake, and living an unhealthy sedentary lifestyle also contribute significantly to the problem.

Emotional stress/distress from a variety of causes often produces overeating, overweight, and obesity. For many people, food has become their "tranquilizer" and their unhealthy way of dealing with the "emotional problems of everyday living" and "civilization and its discontents".

Environmental causes need to be considered as major determinants of overweight and obesity in most cases, especially in the United States and the rest of the Western World. These factors are related primarily to an unhealthy lifestyle excessive food/calorie intake, and lack of physical activity/ exercise. An overabundance of palatable, calorie-dense foods, and aggressive and sophisticated food marketing by the food industry and mass media, supermarkets and restaurants all contribute to the overweight and obesity problem. Large food portions, snacks and desserts at home and eating large meals in restaurants and at social events, all promote excessive caloric consumption.

Sociocultural traditions also tend to promote overeating and consumption of certain high-calorie foods. Levels of physical activity often prove to be inadequate to offset extra food/calorie consumption. Sedentary lifestyle consisting of sitting at work, or in traffic, on the couch, in front of a television set, radio, or a computer for long periods of time all contribute to the overweight, obesity and health-related complications problems.

Once an individual's daily lifestyle becomes biased towards promoting and perpetuating overweight and obesity, increased levels of knowledge, motivation, and behavior management skills and lifestyle changes are required to overcome the problems(s). Much education and counseling become necessary for an individual to acquire the necessary knowledge and skills to succeed in the prevention of overweight and obesity.

For additional information, consult:
National Heart, Lung, and Blood Institute
* Report on: *Guidelines on Overweight and Obesity: Electronic Textbook: Environment*
  http://www.nhlbi.nih.gov/guidelines/obesity/e_txtbk/ratnl/24htm
* Report on: *Guidelines on Overweight and Obesity: Electronic Textbook: Genetic Influence in the Development of Overweight and Obesity*
  http://www.nhlbi.nih.gov/guidelines/obesity/e_txtbk/ratnl/25htm

4.0 Prevention

4.1 Introduction

Prevention of overweight, obesity and health-related complications involves:

- adopting a healthy lifestyle
- fostering good nutrition and eating habits
- engaging in daily physical activity/exercise
- behavior modification
- achieving/maintaining normal body weight

4.2   Healthy Lifestyle

Basic principles to consider for a healthy lifestyle* include:
- alcohol sparingly or not at all
- autograph your work in excellence
- be a friend to many and have many friends
- believe and have confidence in yourself
- choose a physician and health care facility prudently
- communicate effectively with all
- comprehensive annual check-up/follow up
- develop and maintain a rich and full spiritual life
- discover your potential in life
- do no intentional harm to anyone
- do not procrastinate: learn how to make decisions
- drugs: no illegal drugs, use prescription drugs as directed
- eat in healthy and nutritionally sound ways
- exercise, become physically active and fit
- follow safety rules and avoid injuries
- follow your bliss
- have a laudable purpose in life
- have faith and hope in the future
- maintain good family relationships
- make the world a better place
- moderation in living, working and playing
- practice good health habits
- regular and restful daily sleep

- relaxation and stress reduction daily
- rest regularly
- safe and effective health practices
- set and accomplish goals
- strive for emotional well-being and control
- take charge, control and responsibility for your health and life
- tobacco: refrain from use
- weight: attain and maintain ideal weight

*adopted from Web Information Resource Guide by Eugene A. DeFelice, M.D., published by Author's Choice Press, iuniverse.com, August 2001

For additional information on a healthy lifestyle, consult:
- American Academy of Family Physicians—http://www.aafp.org
- American Medical Association—http://www.ama-assn.org
- Heathfinder.Gov—http://www.healthfinder.gov

Chronic diseases, including overweight and obesity, account for 7 out of every 10 deaths, and for more than 60% of medical care expenditures in the US. In addition, the prolonged illness and disability, associated with many chronic diseases, decrease the quality of life for millions of Americans, and overweight and obesity and health-related complications are no exception to this.

Much of the chronic disease burden in the US is preventable with available means. Physical inactivity and unhealthy eating practices contribute to overweight, obesity and health-related complications such as cardiovascular disease, type 2 non-insulin dependent diabetes mellitus, and cancer. Overweight and obesity now are regarded as responsible for well over 300,000 deaths each year, and only tobacco use is responsible for more preventable deaths in the US each year. People who engage in a healthy lifestyle, and avoid risks for overweight and obesity can expect to live a healthier, happier, and longer life.

For example, regular physical activity/exercise is reported to substantially reduce the risk of dying from heart disease, colon and prostate cancer, diabetes, and high blood pressure, etc. Physical activity/exercise also helps to control weight, contribute to healthy bones, improve fitness and mobility, reduce falls and fractures especially among the elderly, relieve pain of arthritis, and lessen anxiety and depression often associated with chronic diseases. It also is associated with less hospitalizations, physician visits, and prescription medication utilization. Moreover, physical activity/exercise need not be strenuous to be beneficial. People of all ages benefit from moderate physical activity/exercise such as walking five or more times a week for 30-60 minutes or more.

Good nutrition lowers the risk for many chronic diseases including overweight and obesity, cardiovascular disease, stroke, some types of cancer and diabetes, etc. For example, for at least 10 million Americans at risk for type 2 diabetes, proper nutrition and physical activity can sharply lower their chances of getting the disease.

The National Center for Chronic Disease Prevention and Health Promotion (NCCDPHP) provides a key report on "*Physical Activity and Good Nutrition: Essential Elements to Prevent Chronic Diseases and Obesity*" at: http://www.cdc.gov/nccdphp.dnpa/dnpaaag.htm.

"*Recommended Strategies to Prevent Chronic Diseases and Obesity*" report is available at:
http://www.cdc.gov/nccdphp/dnpa/obesity/recommendations.htm

"Partnership for a Healthy Weight Management" report provides strategies for achieving and maintaining a healthy weight and is available at: http://www.consumer.gov

A guide for promoting moderate physical activity entitled *"Ready, Set, Its Everywhere You Go"* (http://www.cdc.gov/nccdphp/dnpa/readyset/index.htm.) helps show adults how easy it is to fit physical activity into their busy schedule by just choosing the strategies, programs, event ideas and tools discussed that best fit your needs.

The NCCDPHP's *"Physical Activity Evaluation Handbook"*, (http://www.cdc.gov/nccdphp/dnpa/physical/handbook/index.htm) is a key resource that outlines the 6 basic steps of a physical activity program and illustrates each step with examples. Appendices provide information about physical activity indicators, practical case studies, and additional evaluation resources.

The *"Physical Activity Recommendations"* report (http://www.cdc.gov/nccdphp/dnpa/physical/recommendations.htm) provides health behavior changes tailored to an individual's specific interest and readiness to make required changes in physical activity habits. It is a guide to behavioral skills such as goal setting, building social support, self-rewards, problem solving, and relapse prevention assisting individuals in learning to incorporate physical activity into their daily routines.

To help you plan how to fit physical activity into your day at home, work, or elsewhere, and assist you in getting started, NCCDPHP suggests that:
- walking be included as an integral part of your daily life
- a brisk walk also should be included in your daily activities at least 5-7 days per week. Gradually work up to a brisk 3-mile a day walk

which can be completed in 1, 2 or 3 equally divided intervals. Walking should be considered a great way to start the day off. Bring your dog, a friend, or family member along.

- you take the stairs at work instead of the elevator—at least part of the way, if not the entire way
- physical activity also be incorporated into your weekends, days off, and holidays as well by:
  - getting up and going out doors somewhere such as park, hiking, etc
  - walking when doing errands, shopping, etc, whenever possible
  - making weekend, days off, and holiday walks/exercise a family affair
  - mowing the grass, raking the leaves, gardening, and cleaning the car, garage, cellar, attic and residence should become part of your day's physical activities. Active chores provide a great opportunity to "kill two birds with one stone" by combining moderate-intensity physical activity with getting the chores done at the same time.

"*Promoting Active Lifestyle Among Older Adults*" report provides information on the primary and secondary benefits of physical activity in preventing overweight, obesity and health-related complications in the elderly. It can be found at:
http://www.cdc.gov/nccdphp/dnpa/physical/lifestyles.htm

"*National Blueprint: Increasing Physical Activity Among Adults 50 and Older*" report details 60 specific recommendations for achieving the public health goal of a more physically active older population to reduce the impact of overweight, obesity and health-related complications. It can be found at:
http://www.cdc.gov/nccdphp/dnpa/press/blueprint.htm

"*Promoting Better School Health for Young People*" report highlights the fact that American's children are, in a large measure, inactive, unfit and increasingly overweight or obese. This report outlines 8 strategies to promote health and reduce overweight and obesity through lifelong participation in enjoyable and safe lifestyle changes. It is available at: http://www.cdc.nccdphp/dash/about/comprehensive_ed.htm

Despite common knowledge that exercise is healthful in preventing overweight, obesity and health-related complications, more than 60% of American adults are not regularly physically active, and 25% of the adult population are not active at all. "*Healthy People 2010*" program (http://www.health.gov/healthypeople) for the nation's health recognizes the importance of physical activity/exercise, and has included this in their goals.

Dietary Guidelines for Americans (http://www.cdc.gov/nccdphp/sgr/summ.htm) recommends good nutrition and physical activity/exercise for all.

4.3   Aim for a Healthy Weight

4.3.1 Introduction

Everyone should aim for a healthy weight. The NIH Expert Panel on Identification, Evaluation and Treatment of Overweight and Obesity in Adults recommends:
*   weight loss to lower:
    *   elevated blood pressure in overweight and obese individuals with high blood pressure
    *   increased levels of total cholesterol, LDL cholesterol, and triglycerides, and to raise low levels of HDL cholesterol in overweight and obese individuals with dyslipidemia

- abnormal blood glucose and insulin levels in overweight and obese individuals especially those with overt type 2 diabetes mellitus
- BMI to be used to:
    - assess overweight and obesity. However, body weight alone can be used to follow weight loss, and to determine effectiveness of therapy
    - classify overweight and obesity, and to estimate relative risk of disease complications compared to normal weight
- waist circumference as a measure to assess abdominal fat content of the body.
- initial goal of weight loss therapy should be to reduce body weight by about 10% from baseline (weight at start of treatment). If successful, further weight loss can be attempted.
- weight loss should be targeted at 1-2 pounds per week for a period of at least 6 months with subsequent strategy based on the amount of weight lost.
- low calorie, low fat diet should be used for weight loss in overweight and obese individuals. Reducing fat as part of the low calorie diet is a practical way to reduce calories.
- reducing dietary fat alone without reducing calories is not sufficient for weight loss. However, reducing dietary fat along with reducing dietary carbohydrates helps to reduce calories
- diet individually planned to create a deficit of 500-1000 calories/day should be an integral part of any program
- physical activity should be included as part of a comprehensive weight loss or weight control program because it: 1) modestly contributes to weight loss in overweight and obese adults, 2) may help decrease abdominal fat, 3) increases cardio-respiratory fitness, and 4) helps with maintenance of weight loss.
- moderate levels of physical activity 3-5 days a week are encouraged initially. All adults should set a long-term goal to accumulate at

least 30-60 minutes of moderate-intensity physical activity/exercise on most, if not all days of the week.

- a combination of a reduced calorie diet and increased physical activity is recommended since it produces weight loss that may also result in decreases in abdominal fat and increases in cardio-respiratory fitness.
- behavior therapy is a useful adjunct when incorporated into treatment for weight loss and weight maintenance.
- weight loss and weight maintenance therapy should employ the combination of a low calorie/low fat diet, increased physical activity, and behavior modification therapy
- after successful weight loss, the likelihood of weight loss maintenance is enhanced by a program consisting of diet, physical activity/exercise, and behavior modification that should be continued indefinitely. Drug therapy can also be used to enhance weight loss results. However, drug safety and efficacy beyond 1 year of total treatment have not been established.
- a weight maintenance program should be a priority after the initial 6 months of weight loss therapy if further progress is not anticipated.

For additional information consult:
National Heart, Lung and Blood institute
- Report on: *Aim for a healthy weight: Key Recommendations*
  http://www.nhlbi.nih.gov/health/public/heart/obsity/lose-wt/recommend.htm
- Report on: *Selecting a Weight Loss Program*
  http://www.nhlbi.nih.gov/health/public/heart/obesity/lose-wt/wtl_prog.htm

4.3.2 Unhealthy Body Weight/Health Risk

An unhealthy body weight is associated with disease risks relative to BMI and waist circumference as indicated in Table III below:

Table III—BMI, Waist Circumference and Medical Risk

Weight Class	BMI	Obesity Class	Waist Circumference	
			Group A* Risk	Group B** Risk
Normal	18.5-24.9	—	—	—
Overweight	25.0-29.9	—	Increased	High
Obesity	30.0-34.9	I	High	Very High
	35.0-39.9	II	Very High	Very High
Extreme Obesity	40.0+	III	Extremely High	Extremely High

*Men—40 inches (102 cm) or less, Women—35 inches (88 cm) or less
**Men—greater than 40 inches (102 cm), Women—greater than 35 inches (88cm)

Disease risk in table above is for type 2 diabetes mellitus, and cardiovascular disease.
Reference: http://www.nhlbi.nih.gov/health/public/heart/obesity/lose_wt/bmi_dis.htm

Recent studies indicate that being overweight, even obese by BMI standards, isn't as unhealthy as being sedentary, or largely inactive. In a large study of some 22,000 men over a period of 8 years, the lean and unfit, as measured by treadmill performance, were found to be twice as likely to die as the fit, including the obese fit. Other studies appear to support the idea that diet alone is not the answer for overweight and obese individuals. A healthful diet plus physical activity/exercise is considered to be more appropriate and effective.

While 30-60 minutes or more of moderate daily exercise (such as a brisk 3 mile walk) has been shown to reduce health-related complications of overweight and obesity regardless of whether the activity reduces weight, available evidence appears to indicate that the mitigating effect on complications is much greater in those who do lose significant weight.

For additional information, consult:

National Heart, Lung and Blood Institute
• Report on: *Assessing Your Risk*
  http://www.nhlbi.nih.gov/health/public/heart/obesity/lose_wt/risk.htm
• Report on: *Aim for a Healthy Weight: Key Recommendations*
  http://www.nhlbi.nih.gov/health/public/heart/obesity/lose_wt/recommen.htm

4.4 Diet Controversy

4.4.1 Overview

Individuals gain weight by burning less, lose weight by burning more, and maintain normal weight by burning essentially the same number of calories as consumed. Eating fewer calories means consuming less food, and burning more calories necessitates becoming more physically active/exercising. Weight gain is caused by consumption of an excess of total calories, whether fat or carbohydrate, over expenditure. Thus, the key to prevention of overweight and obesity remains a healthy combination of physical activity/exercise and caloric restriction. Calories do count.

There is little controversy over the physical activity/exercise side of the equation for weight control. However, there appears to be recent controversy over the three general classes of diets for weight control and the prevention of overweight, obesity and health-related complication. These three general classes of diet are: 1) high-fat with essentially no calorie restriction, 2) low to moderate fat with calorie restriction, and 3) very low fat with no calorie restriction.

Little doubt exists that one can control their body weight, prevent weight gain, or lose weight on most diets over the short term regardless of class of diet used. However, the question remains regarding which diet is most effective and safe for a given individual or patient population over the long haul for the healthiest, longest life. Unfortunately, conclusive answers to these questions are largely lacking in the present state of our knowledge. Thus, diet choice is largely empirical although some knowledge exists upon which to base decisions.

4.4.2 Atkins' High Fat Diet

The so-called "diet revolution" championed by Dr. Robert C. Atkins has stirred up the controversy over which diet is best for Americans to control their weight or lose it when needed. This diet is designed not to limit caloric intake or the amount of fat (e.g. from meat, eggs, cheese, etc) that one consumes. It is based on the premise that high fat foods not only digest more slowly but also make one feel satisfied longer, thus limiting food intake. Being very low in carbohydrates, the Atkins' diet causes the body to manufacture ketones that suppress hunger further making it easier to adhere to over the short as well as the long term. In addition, the diet is reported to preserve lean body mass, sparing muscle loss, and decreasing blood glucose and insulin levels.

The Atkins' Diet is reported to be relatively easy to follow and adhere to, and reasonably effective in maintaining normal weight or promoting weight loss in those overweight. However, long-term effectiveness and safety remain to be demonstrated in large-scale well-controlled clinical trials.

On the negative side, there appears to be an increased risk of kidney stones in patients using the Atkins' Diet. Also, high fat diets are reported to decrease the flow of blood to the heart muscle compromising function accordingly, especially in susceptible people with coronary artery disease. Diets high in saturated fat also raise serum cholesterol and this carries a risk of coronary heart disease and myocardial infarction.

In contrast, diets rich in fruits and vegetables, and low to moderate in protein and fat, have been shown to prevent or ameliorate high blood pressure, heart disease, type 2 diabetes mellitus, and reduce the risk of some cancers. Decreasing saturated fat in the diet also reduces coronary heart disease by 24%.

The typical Atkins' Diet is lacking in adequate calcium, B vitamins, and vitamins A, C, and D, as well as antioxidants that may help prevent cardiovascular disease and slow the aging process, and calcium. Too much animal protein in such a diet from meats may even lead to leaching of calcium from bone, increasing the risk of osteopenia, osteoporosis, and fractures. Patients on the Atkins' Diet require supplements of deficient nutrients to avoid such complications.

Current interest in the Atkins' Diet appears to be due to claims that low to moderate, and very low fat diets may be more difficult to adhere to, or not work as effectively in weight maintenance and weight loss. However, such claims have not been demonstrated to be true in large-scale well-controlled clinical trials to date.

In short, comparative clinical trials are needed to demonstrate conclusively just how effective and safe the Atkins' Diet is for the prevention of overweight, obesity and health-related complications. While such clinical trials are reported to be planned or underway now, it will be some time before results are available.

For additional information, consult: http://www.atkinscenter.com.

4.4.3 Low to Moderate Fat Diet

In the past, a 30% total fat, 10% or less saturated fat, has been considered a low fat diet recommended by US Dietary Guidelines, American Heart Association and National Cholesterol Guidelines for NHLBI. Today, this same diet is called moderate fat.

In contrast to the lack of substantial well-controlled clinical trial evidence for the Atkins' Diet, there are a number of well-designed, randomized controlled clinical trials regarding the efficacy and safety of low to moderate fat diets showing that reducing dietary fat is a practical way to reduce calories in the diet and promote normal weight and even desired weight loss as needed.

The National Institutes of Health Diabetes Prevention Program has provided evidence that a diet limiting fats to 25% of total calories, combined with exercise, produces significant sustained weight loss and keeps it off for at least 4 years in most people evaluated. In addition, such a diet is reported to significantly cut the risk of developing type 2 diabetes mellitus by almost 60%.

Clinical studies show that the more closely one follows a reduced calorie, low to moderate (25% to 30%) fat diet, the more their heart disease and high blood pressure improves. And individuals who consume a reduced calorie, low to moderate fat diet, appear to lose about as much weight as seen with the Atkins' Diet without worsening of cardiovascular disease risk.

A large USDA *Continuing Survey of Food Intake by Individuals* (10,000 randomly selected and interviewed at home), concerning their eating habits, found that those who eat a low to moderate fat diet are more likely to weigh less and consume on average 200 to 300 few calories, than those who eat a high-fat diet.

Available evidence indicates that a 10% reduction in dietary fat alone is associated with a weight loss of a quarter of a pound per week or 13 pounds per year. And, those who succeed at losing desired weight and keeping it off, generally follow a low to moderate fat diet, limit food/caloric intake, and avail themselves of an abundance of physical activity/exercise

Finally, while one maintains normal weight, or loses weight on a high protein, high fat diet due to eating fewer simple carbohydrates, one apparently can lose as much weight by eating fewer simple carbohydrates and less fat. Thus, it appears that a calorie restricted, low to moderate fat diet apparently remains the choice for prevention of weight gain, or the treatment of overweight, obesity and health-related complications for most people until proven otherwise.

4.4.4 Dr. Ornish's Very Low Fat Diet

The Ornish diet is at the other extreme of the three classes of the diet controversy. With this diet, it is reported that you can eat all you want providing foods consumed are very low in fat and high in fiber. The fiber content is designed to fill you up, reduce hunger/desire to eat, and thus curtail food/calorie intake.

Available evidence appears to indicate that the longer one follows such a very low fat, whole foods diet (complex carbohydrates such as unrefined whole-wheat bread, brown rice, fruits, vegetables, beans, etc.) the healthier one apparently becomes. For example, in patients on such a diet, angina pectoris is reported to be decreased by over 90% and cholesterol levels by 40% without the use of medications. Also, patients needing coronary bypass surgery or angioplasty apparently are able to avoid these procedures by following Dr. Ornish's very low fat diet.

While Dr. Ornish's diet was originally designed mainly for people with heart disease—some of whom apparently were able to reverse the course of their disease for the better—it is now also considered to be useful for prevention of overweight, obesity and health-related complications such as cardiovascular disease, high blood pressure, stroke, type 2 diabetes mellitus, etc.

Whether Dr. Ornish's very low fat diet eventually will prove to be the most desirable for the prevention and/or treatment of overweight, obesity and health-related complications remains to be established in further large-scale well-controlled clinical trials in comparison with other diets. Some such trials are expected to be completed in coming years.

For additional information, consult:
http://www.ornish.com

4.5   Dietary Guidelines for Healthy Adults

The US Department of Agriculture has published *Dietary Guidelines for Americans* which can be found at: http://www.nal.usda.gov/fnic/dga/dguide95.html.

Anyone using these USDA Guidelines should bear in mind that calories do count, caloric intake should balance expenditure for weight maintenance, and refined (simple) carbohydrates (sugars) are not as good for you as complex ones. To maintain normal weight and prevent overweight and obesity, restriction of fat and calories consumed in the diet is a necessity. One must adjust and balance the amount of energy in the food consumed with the amount of energy the body uses over time in order to maintain "normal" weight. And, physical activity/exercise remain key/important ways to burn calories.

Dietary Guidelines for Healthy American Adults recommended by the American Heart Association (AHA) are in essential agreement with the USDA Guidelines and are designed to:
*   help one achieve and maintain a healthy eating pattern and body weight
*   reduce the risk of cardiovascular disease, type 2 diabetes mellitus, bone loss, some forms of cancer, and other chronic health problems

These AHA Dietary Guidelines generally recommend that one:
*   balance levels of caloric intake and physical activity/exercise to control weight
*   eat a nutritionally sound diet consisting of a variety of foods
*   eat 5 or more servings per day of a variety of fruits and vegetables
*   consume 6 or more servings per day of a variety of grain products, principally whole grains

- reduce total calories from saturated fat
- limit food high in saturated fat, trans fat and/or cholesterol, and those high in calories or low in nutrition such as soft drinks, and candy/snacks that are high in sugar
- eat at least two servings of fish per week
- consume no more than 2400 milligrams of sodium,
- drink no more than 1 to 2 ounces of alcohol containing beverages per day

For additional information and details consult:
http://www.americanheart.org, and search "dietary guidelines".

4.6   Basal Metabolic Rate/Basal Energy Expenditure

Basal metabolic rate (BMR) or basal energy expenditure (BEE) is the estimated amount of energy the body requires on a daily basis in order to carry out its basic functions at rest.

BMR or BEE may be estimated by the equation recommended by Miffen et al* as follows:

BMR=[9.99 x weight in kilograms]+[6.25 x height in centimeters]—[4.92 x age in years]+[1.66 x sex, where male=1 and female=0]—161

*Mifflin et al. A new predictive equation for resting energy expenditure in healthy individuals. Am. J. Clin. Nutrition 51: 241-247, 1990.

Alternatively, one may use the Harris-Benedict equation to estimate BMR as follows:

BMR (males)=66+[13.7 x weight in kilograms}+[5.0 x height in centimeters]—[6.8 x age in years].

BMR (females)=655+[9.5 x weight in kilograms]+[1.8 x height in centimeters—[4.7 x age in years]

These equations take into account height, weight, age and sex in estimating BMR, and are considered to be more accurate than other methods.

A simpler but less accurate estimate of BMR involves multiplying body weight in pounds by 10. Thus, if one weight 165 pounds for example, BMR would be around 1,650 calories just to maintain body weight at rest.

Regardless of the method used to estimate BMR one needs to multiply this figure by an activity level factor as follows:

Activity Level   Activity Level Factor

1. Low (sedentary)   1.3
2. Intermediate (some regular exercise)   1.5
3. High (regular physical activity/exercise
   or a physically demanding job)   1.7

BMR estimate plus added calories per activity level factor provides an estimate for daily caloric intake necessary to maintain stable body weight.

The American Heart Association advocates another simple method for estimating total daily caloric energy expenditure. AHA recommends multiplying the number of pounds one weighs by 15 calories. The figure obtained by this method then becomes the estimated number of calories needed to be consumed in one day if one is moderately active in order to maintain stable body weight. However, if one is not very physically active, weight should be multiplied by 13 calories because less-active individuals burn fewer calories.

Figures obtained by any of the above methods should be considered only as rough estimates at best, and caloric intake versus expenditure needs to be adjusted periodically (e.g., monthly) for satisfactory weight control over time.

In addition, one needs to keep in mind that certain conditions may also increase or decrease energy expenditure. For example, energy expenditure is increased with fever by 13% for each degree Centigrade above normal, by 10-100% in patients with hyperthyroidism, and 40-100% in patients with trauma. Those with other conditions also may have altered daily caloric expenditure accordingly. In contrast, patients with malabsorption may absorb as few as 25% of ingested calories and have a corresponding caloric deficit.

For additional information on prevention, consult:

National Heart, Lung, and Blood Institute
http://www.nhlbi.nih.gov/guidleins/obesity/e_txtbk/ratnl/23.htm

Health.gov/Nutrition and Your Health: Dietary Guidelines
http://www.health.gov/dietaryguidelines

National Center for Chronic Disease Prevention
http://www.cdc.gov/nccdphp/dnpa

Just Move.org
http://www.justmove.org

Shape Up America
http://www.shapeup.org

President's Council on Physical Fitness and Sports
http://www.fitness.gov

5. Health Complications

5.1 Introduction

Overweight and obese individuals remain at significant increased risk for serious health complications, and even premature death. Complications/mortality rates are directly related to weight increase above normal for height and age. However, it needs to be recognized that not all overweight or obese individuals develop such health complications. Reasons for this may be related to degree of cardiovascular and muscular fitness, locations of fat on the body and body fat composition, and other factors that may play a role.

In men, 50% or greater above normal weight, mortality rates are increased approximately two fold, five fold for diabetics and four fold in those with digestive tract disease. In females with the same percentage weight gain over normal, morality is increased two fold, while those with diabetes mortality is increased eight fold, and three fold in those with digestive tract disease. Overweight people of both sexes, especially young overweight individuals, tend to die significantly sooner than their lean contemporaries. While obesity is an important factor in itself, most mortality appears to be associated with complications.

Key complications associated with overweight and obesity include one or more of the following:

- cardiovascular disease
  - coronary heart disease/angina pectoris
  - myocardial infarction
  - hypertension (high blood pressure)
  - congestive heart failure
  - cardiomyopathy
  - dyslipidemia
  - stroke
  - peripheral vascular disease
- diabetes mellitus (type 2, non insulin-dependent)
  - hyperinsulinemia
  - insulin resistance
  - glucose intolerance
- Syndrome X (Metabolic Syndrome X)
- cancer
- gallbladder disease
  - cholelithiasis (gallstones)
  - cholecystitis (infection, inflammation)
- osteoarthritis (degenerative arthritis)
- gout
  - gouty arthritis
  - uric acid kidney stones (nephrolithiasis)
- sleep apnea
- hiatus hernia
- female reproductive system disorders
- psychological disorders
- premature death
- other complications

5.2 Cardiovascular disease

Overweight and obesity significantly increase the risk of coronary heart disease, angina pectoris, myocardial infarction, congestive heart failure, cardiomyopathy, high blood pressure, stroke, peripheral vascular disease and dyslipidemias. Large waist circumference or high waist-to-hip ratio are significant cardiovascular risk factors.

Dyslipidemia (combinations of high blood cholesterol and/or, triglycerides, high LDL (low density lipoprotein) cholesterol, and low HDL (high density lipoprotein) cholesterol) further dispose individuals to cardiovascular disease complications.

Up to two thirds of overweight/obese individuals suffer from hypertension (high blood pressure). Studies show a direct relationship between android or central obesity and hypertension. And, recent evidence suggests that an obesity gene may be involved in those individuals having both hypertension and obesity.

Stroke and peripheral vascular disease also are a not uncommon complications especially in patients with hypertension, and a high waist-to-hip ratio.

Overweight/obese individuals not uncommonly suffer from Syndrome X (Metabolic Syndrome X) which puts them at high risk for coronary heart disease and type 2 diabetes mellitus.

Cardiomyopathy, fatty infiltration of the heart, appears to be closely related to the duration of obesity. This complication is reported to occur more commonly in those individuals who have been obese for 10 or more years.

The death rate from cardiovascular disease is reported to be around 50% higher for those who are moderately obese and 90% higher for those with severe obesity.

Diet, exercise, weight loss, lifestyle changes and certain medications significantly reduce the development of such complications and premature death.

5.3   Diabetes Mellitus

Overweight and obesity increase the demand for insulin and are associated with hyperinsulinemia, insulin resistance, and type 2 diabetes mellitus (non insulin-dependent). High waist-to-hip ratio, increased waist circumference, insulin resistance, dyslipidemia, poor diet, physical inactivity, sedentary lifestyle, and Syndrome X (Metabolic Syndrome X) are all risk factors for the development of type 2 diabetes mellitus.

Type 2 diabetes mellitus now affects more than 16 million people in the US. It is regarded as the main cause of kidney failure, limb amputations, new onset blindness in adults, and a major cause of cardiovascular disease, hypertension, peripheral vascular disease, and stroke. Type 2 diabetes mellitus accounts for up to 95% of all diabetes cases in the US. It is strongly associated with overweight and obesity (over 80% are overweight or obese), inactivity, family history of diabetes, and racial, ethnic and socioeconomic background. Compared to whites, black adults are reported to have a 60% higher rate of type 2 diabetes mellitus while Hispanic adults have a 90% higher rate.

The prevalence of type 2 diabetes mellitus in the US has tripled in the last 30 years and much of this increase is reported to be due to the dramatic upswing of overweight and obesity. Individuals with a BMI of 30 or greater have at least a five-fold greater risk of type 2 diabetes compared with those with a normal BMI.

A recent large USA clinical study indicates 10 million or more Americans, at high risk for type 2 diabetes, can sharply lower their chances for developing diabetes by almost 60% with diet, exercise and weight loss. Other clinical studies in China and Finland also have shown that diet, exercise, and weight loss can significantly delay development of type 2 diabetes mellitus.

5.4   Syndrome X (Metabolic Syndrome X)

A significant number of overweight/obese individuals have a cluster of key risk factors that make them especially prone to develop coronary heart disease and "heart attacks". This cluster of risk factors is referred to as Syndrome X or Metabolic Syndrome X. The modifier "metabolic" is used to differentiate this condition from another so-called "cardiac syndrome x" or "chest pain syndrome x"—in which a patient complains of angina pectoris-like chest pain in the absence of demonstrable evidence of coronary heart disease. Whether or not these disorders are related in any way remains to be determined.

Recognition of Syndrome X in overweight/obese individuals is particularly important since it carries a high risk for cardiovascular disease complications and premature death.

Syndrome X risk factors include:
*   android or central body obesity (larger than normal waist circumference and excessive fat accumulation in the abdominal region)
*   essential hypertension

- dyslipidemia—primarily high blood triglycerides, low HDL (high density lipoprotein) cholesterol, and high LDL (low density lipoprotein) cholesterol
- hyperinsulinemia (high blood insulin levels)
- insulin resistance
- glucose intolerance
- blood clotting abnormalities

Some individuals with Syndrome X have primarily hypertension, hyperinsulinemia, and insulin-resistance but do not have type 2 diabetes mellitus. Others may have principally hypertension and insulin-resistance, and compensate by producing increased amounts of insulin (hyperinsulinemia). And still others may have primarily hyperinsulinemia with normal blood glucose levels. Only a minority of patients has all risk factors present. Additional research needs to be done to clarify the relationship and roles played among the various risk factors for Syndrome X and their consequences.

Insulin resistance however appears to be a key abnormality involved in most cases of Syndrome X. This insulin resistance eventually appears to lead to type 2 diabetes mellitus and cardiovascular complications.

Syndrome X treatment is empirical at this time. Weight loss, diet, and exercise appear to offer benefit in many cases. Medications such as metformin may be used to reduce insulin resistance. Treatment may be aimed at each of the individual risk factors such as hyperlipidemia, hypertension, and abnormalities of blood clotting, etc.

5.5   Cancer

Cancer mortality rates are increased significantly in obese females— uterus (endometrium/lining)—5.4 times, gallbladder—3.6 times, cervix—2.4 times, ovary—1.6 times, and breast—1.5times. In obese males, cancer mortality rates are increased 1.7 times for the colorectum and 1.3 times for the prostate. Thus, overweight and particularly obesity, are associated in a significant manner with certain types of cancer.

5.6   Gallbladder Disease

Gallstones (cholelithiasis) is reported to occur 3 times more often in obese, compared to non-obese, individuals. Rapid weight loss, and the use of very low calorie diets (VLCD) plus certain drugs (e.g., statins used to treat high blood cholesterol/triglycerides) significantly increase the risk of occurrence of gallstones. Cholecystitis, an infection/inflammation of the gallbladder, is a common complication of gallstones. Both gallstones and cholecystitis may require surgical intervention.

5.7   Osteoarthritis (Degenerative Arthritis)

Degenerative arthritis of the spine, hip and knees—and the pain, discomfort, and decreased mobility resulting, increases with increasing weight in overweight and obese individuals especially as they age. Weight reduction, diet, exercise, and lifestyle changes are known to mitigate these problems.

5.8   Gout

Gout (increased blood uric acid levels), gouty arthritis, and uric acid kidney stones not uncommonly are complications of overweight and obesity. Weight reduction, lifestyle changes, diet and exercise plus medication(s) are essential for prevention and treatment.

5.9   Hiatus Hernia

Hiatus hernia occurs, particularly in obese individuals, when the stomach protrudes (herniates) through the diaphragm, into the chest cavity through an enlarged opening compressing the stomach, lungs and heart, compromising their function. When particularly symptomatic, hiatus hernia may require significant weight loss and surgical correction.

5.10   Sleep Apnea

Obesity is regarded as a principal cause in up to two-thirds of patients diagnosed with sleep apnea. The sleep apnea syndrome occurs when breathing is obstructed, particularly during sleep, because of collapse of the upper airway due to obesity—causing the patient to awaken repeatedly during the night—resulting in failing to obtain a restful night's sleep. Daytime sleepiness occurs as a result, and this leads to impaired and decreased performance during the day. The sleep apnea syndrome is associated with the risk of accidents (e.g., home, auto, work, etc) and cardiovascular and cerebrovascular disease. Appropriate weight reduction is essential. The Pickwickian Syndrome (severe advanced sleep apnea syndrome) is considered a medical emergency because it is frequently fatal.

5.11   Female Reproductive Disorders

Reproductive disorders tend to occur primarily in females with android or central obesity, and are more common in women with greater degrees if overweight and obesity. Included are such disorders as early menarche, hirsuitism, failure to ovulate or to menstruate, decreased fertility, and delayed menopause. Significant weight loss and its maintenance are necessary for improvement.

5.12   Psychological Disorders

Overweight and obesity frequently are associated with stress/distress, anxiety, depression, and eating disorder(s). These factors need to be taken into consideration not only as possible psychological complications but also in prevention and treatment of overweight and obese individuals. Counseling, behavior modification, lifestyle changes are basic to the management of these disorders.

5.13   Premature Death

The risk of dying prematurely from overweight and obesity increases with increasing body weight and BMI. Premature death is particularly notable in the obese—especially in the moderately to severely obese individuals.

5.14   Other Complications

Pregnancy, surgical, and other complications occur with increasing frequency in the overweight and obese. Discussion of such is beyond the scope of this book and the reader is referred to the Author's List of Web Resources for such information.

Overweight and obesity now are considered to represent a major serious threat to the health of the United States and the rest of the Western World because they are regarded as accounting for:

- 90-95% of all type 2 diabetes mellitus
- 50-70% of all heart disease
- 70% of gallbladder disease
- 35% of hypertension
- 10% or so of colon, breast, and prostate cancer
- highly significant amount of premature death and disability

As such, overweight and obesity now constitute a major health epidemic of epic proportions.

For additional information on each health complication, consult:

National Institute Diabetes, Digestive and Kidney Diseases
* Report on: *Do You Know the Health Risks of Being Overweight*
  http://www.niddk.nih.gov/health/nutrit/pubs/health.htnn

* Report on: *Diet and Exercise Dramatically Delay Type 2 Diabetes: Diabetes Medication Metformin Also Effective*
  http://www.niddk.nih.gov/welcome/releases/8_8_01.htm

American Association of Clinical Endocrinologists (AACE)— American College of Endocrinology (ACE)
* Report on: *AACE/ACE Position Statement Regarding the Prevention Diagnosis, and Treatment of Obesity (1998)*
  http://www.aace.com/college (search AACE Obesity Position Statement)

Medlineplus
http://www.nlm.nih.gov/medlineplus

National Institutes of health
http://www.health.nih.gov

Google
http://www.google.com

WebMD
http://www.webmd.com

6.   Diagnosis

Diagnosis of overweight/obesity is based on an assessment of:
- patient and family history
- clinical examination and body measurements
- battery of appropriate laboratory tests
- degree and type of overweight/obesity
- assessment of health risks/complications
- mental health status

Such assessments are usually made in cases of obesity but not necessarily in all overweight patients.

Factors of importance in the patient's history to be assessed include such things as:
- eating habits and diet
- degree of physical activity/exercise
- presence of stress factors and psychological disorders
- types of, and results of, previous weight loss attempts
- weight history (maximum, minimum, changes, current)
- drug and alcohol use and degree of consumption
- weight loss medication use and results
- level of motivation to follow recommended treatment

Basic laboratory tests may include such things as:
- blood
  - lipid profile (e.g., cholesterol, triglycerides, LDL, HDL, etc)
  - fasting blood sugar and insulin levels regarding diabetes
  - battery of blood chemistries including uric acid
- routine urine analysis

Other laboratory tests may be needed to assess complications and uncommon causes of overweight/obesity such as hypothyroidism (thyroid function tests), Cushing's syndrome (cortisol levels), polycystic ovary syndrome, (hormone levels) etc. Discussion of such is beyond the scope of this book and will not be considered further.

At the present time, body measurements such as weight (using healthy weight ranges for men and women), waist-to-hip ratio, waist circumference, body mass index and body fat distribution are the principal means used in assessing and classifying overweight and obesity. All these clinical methods as well as others may be used, in combination with clinical evaluation to assess overweight and obesity, degree of body fat and its distribution, and medical risks involved.

The degree and class of overweight/obesity and body fat distribution usually is assessed by means of the BMI (body mass index), body fat skin caliper, WHR (waist-to-hip ratio), and visually by clinical examination/evaluation.

BMI is used because it correlates well with total body fat and health risk. However, it does not indicate the distribution of body fat. Health risk increases not only as the BMI increases beyond the normal range but also, even more importantly when the patient has at least one health complicating disorder as well.

Waist and hip circumferences, and the ratio of the two, are indicators of the location of body fat. Fat measurements using the body fat skin caliper also provides useful information regarding fat location. Waist circumference correlates well with the amount of abdominal fat that has important implications for the development of type 2 diabetes mellitus and cardiovascular complications. A normogram also may be used to determine the waist-to-hip ratio and health risk associated.

For additional information on the diagnosis of overweight and obesity, consult: *AACE/ACE Position Statement on the Prevention, Diagnosis, and Treatment of Obesity (1998 Revision)* Endocrine Practice, Vol. 4, No., 5, September/October, 1998, pp 297-330. This report is available online at: http://www.aace.com/college. Use the Search site and the topic "obesity" to obtain the report link.

7.   Treatment

7.1   Overview

True success lies in the prevention of overweight, obesity and health-related complications. However, this is not easily accomplished or we would not be facing the present epidemic of overweight and obesity and the consequences. Wide-scaled efforts/programs are being implemented by governmental agencies, health professionals, and others to address the matter of prevention and treatment. Hopefully, these efforts/programs will lead to greater success in the coming years.

Success also can be measured in terms of treatment achieving target weight loss and preventing/lessening health-related complications. It should be recognized that target weight loss may be achieved in many overweight and mild to moderately obese individuals with proper treatment/management. While successful medical treatment remains difficult in the vast majority of severely obese individuals, surgical intervention appears to offer a viable alternative.

For many overweight and mild to moderately obese patients, success needs to be measured in terms of achievable goals, namely a significant beneficial target weight loss of at least 10-15% of body weight along with prevention or improvement in health-related complications such as cardiovascular disease and diabetes, etc. This less than optimal, but fully achievable goal (in most patients), needs to be understood and accepted by both the patient and healthcare provider/physician for the weight loss program to prove to be "successful" and provide a basis for possible further weight loss as needed in the future.

Various strategies may produce this weight loss. However, unless a weight loss maintenance program is put in place once weight is lost, most patients usually regain up to two thirds of the weight lost within the first year, and almost all within 5 years. Reasons for this vary. Failure to continue physical activity/exercise, dieting/caloric restriction, lifestyle changes and behavior modification are some of the reasons. Also, patient demotivation as well as other factors such as a low basal metabolic rate may contribute to the weight regain. In general, however, relapses tend to occur from a complex interaction of biological and psychological factors. Thus, weight loss treatment and maintenance strategy needs to be continued for the long term, and modified as necessary along the way, for success. In any event, the treatment strategy needs to be individualized for optimum results.

When a target weight loss of 10-15% of body weight is achieved and maintained, significant health benefits usually occur. These may include improvement in heart disease, high blood pressure, diabetes mellitus, blood sugar and insulin levels, cholesterol and other lipid levels, sleep apnea, arthritis symptoms, anxiety, depression and mood.

Treatment of overweight, obesity and health-related complications may include: basic medical treatment, drugs/pharmacotherapy, or surgical treatment. For optimal medical treatment, physician supervision may be necessary, particularly in the severely obese and those with medical complications or receiving prescription drugs. However, in some overweight or mild to moderately obese persons without such medical complications or the need for prescription medication, physician supervision/management may not always be necessary.

Regardless of which approach is used, principles underlying successful treatment strategies/programs provide that the patient:
- be treated with sensitivity, respect, and in a professional manner by all concerned
- understand that overweight and obesity are a group of chronic disorders with more than one cause requiring individualized long term treatment similar to that necessary in other chronic diseases
- accept counseling and/or other treatment, as needed for co-existing psychological disorders such as anxiety, depression, stress/distress, behavior modification, and lifestyle changes without which overall treatment is not likely to be very successful
- be afforded informed consent for all aspects of treatment

Some people prefer to lose weight on their own. If one decides to join in any kind of weight loss—or maintenance—program, one needs to consider the following:
- does the program provide counseling to help you change your diet, physical activity, and behavior? The program should teach you how to permanently change lifestyle factors, such as unhealthy diet and physical inactivity that have contributed to weight gain.
- is the staff made up of a variety of qualified health professionals? You need to be evaluated by a physician if you have any health problems, are currently taking any medicine, or plan on taking any medicine, or plan to lose more than 20-30 pounds. If your weight loss plan uses a very low calorie diet (VLCD—a special liquid formula that replaces almost all solid food), a clinical exam/evaluation and follow-up visits by a doctor also are needed.

- is training available on how to deal with times when you may feel stressed and slip back to old habits? Long-term strategies and a support system/group are needed to deal with these problems.
- is attention paid to keeping weight off when lost? A program is needed that teaches skills and techniques to make permanent changes in eating habits and levels of physical activity to prevent weight gain.
- are food choices flexible and suitable to your needs? The program should consider your food likes and dislikes and your lifestyle when your weight loss goals are planned.
- what percentage of people complete this program? Program chosen should have a historical high percentage of successful completions.
- what is the average weight loss among people who finish the program? This figure should at least match your target weight loss goals, and better still, exceed it.
- what percentage of people have problems or side effects? Historically, there should be a low level of problems, and very few you cannot cope with.
- are there fees or costs for additional items used in the program such as prepared meals, dietary supplements, drugs, etc?

Remember, quick weight loss methods usually don't provide lasting results. Weight loss methods that rely on diet aids like drinks, prepackaged foods, or over-the-counter diet pills usually don't work in the long run unless they are part of a comprehensive program. Whether you lose weight on your own or in a group, remember that the most important changes for ultimate success are long term in nature. No matter how much weight you need to lose, modest goals and a slow course likely will increase your chances of losing the weight and keeping it off.

For additional information, consult:

National Heart, Lung and Blood Institute
- Report on: *Selecting a Weight Loss Program*
  http://www.nhlbi.nih.gov/health/public/heart/obesity/lose_wt/
  wtl_prog.htm
- Report on: *Clinical Guidelines on the Identification, Evaluation, and
  Treatment of Overweight and Obesity in Adults*
  http://www.nhblo.nih.gov/guidelines/obesity/ob_home.htm

7.2   Basic Medical Treatment

7.2.1   Introduction

In order to achieve the greatest likelihood of success from a weight loss program, diet, physical activity/exercise, behavior modification and lifestyle changes are essential. These aspects need to be incorporated into a well-designed program supervised by experience professionals to achieve optimal results.

Patient participation in a group therapeutic setting with regular close, continued contact usually achieves the best overall results both in terms of weight loss and its maintenance afterwards.

Experience has demonstrated that basic medical treatment alone can produce weight loss averaging around 1-2 pounds per week on a sustained basis without the aid of prescription drugs or surgical intervention in most cases.

Key components of basic medical treatment are:
- attainable weight loss goal
  Weight loss of 10-15% of body weight is considered reasonable and achievable for most overweight, and mild to moderately obese individuals, in a well-designed and supervised program. Loss averaging

around 1-2 pounds per week after the initial first month should be targeted and expected in most cases.
- regular follow-up contact
This may be done every 1-2 weeks for the first month and at least bimonthly or every month thereafter for:
  - guidance regarding nutrition, exercise and lifestyle changes
  - discussion of risk factors and personal situations
  - mutual sharing and group support
  - fostering a "buddy" relationship in the group
  - physician/health professional monitoring, especially regarding those on very low calorie diets or having medical complications or requiring prescription medications
  - counseling as needed

For additional information, consult:

American Academy of Family Practice
- Report on: *Medical Management of Obesity*
  http://www.aafp.org/afp/20000715/419.htm

7.2.2 Lifestyle Changes

Counseling/education generally is regarded as essential for lifestyle changes and success in any weight loss program. With such, patients are more able to evaluate, understand, and modify their behavior concerning eating practices, necessity of caloric restriction and physical activity/exercise. They are better able to cope with, and modify, the psychological aspects of their overweight, obesity and health-related complications, substantially improving their chances for successful weight loss, etc. Weekly, to bi-monthly or monthly, counseling/education sessions generally are regarded as the norm.

Lifestyle modification programs include such things as self-monitoring, eating stimulus recognition and control, stress management to reduce the use of food to cope with the problems of every day living (e.g., using "food as a tranquilizer"), and certain cognitive-behavioral strategies. Patients are instructed on keeping daily logs/records regarding food intake, physical activity and problems encountered for discussion with a counselor, dietician, or support group to identify lifestyles/behaviors that need to be changed for success. Instruction on "portion control" is essential so one can learn how to recognize more appropriate portion sizes, and caloric content.

Patient instruction/education usually helps one to identify and avoid: 1) environmental factors that may trigger unhealthful eating, particularly at cafeteria or buffet restaurants, traveling, or snacking between meals, and 2) inactivity especially such as may occur during weekends, in front of the TV, and during holidays. Counseling/education and group support sessions teach patients ways to modify or avoid such behaviors.

Stress management is particularly important for those with concomitant psychological disorders, or ones with more serious medical complications such as cardiovascular disease or diabetes. Stress reduction may be accomplished with medication, relaxation techniques, meditation, and with regular physical activity/exercise. These measures enhance coping and reduce the adverse effects of stressful internal and environmental stimuli.

Cognitive behavioral techniques such as the regular use of imagery conditioning or positive self-statements also may be employed. Patients may be instructed to see themselves as losing weight, being thin, and eating, dieting, exercising properly and losing weight, etc. This helps to change an individual's attitudes and beliefs about body image and expectations for the better as well as help bring about better compliance and results.

Support groups are used to help the patient achieve necessary lifestyle changes and weight loss as well as play an important role in maintaining weight loss.

The published literature indicates that results from weight management programs conducted by non-physicians (e.g., dieticians, nutritionists, nurse practitioners, etc) may compare favorably to those supervised by physicians, and may be considered as an alternative to physician supervised programs, providing the individual does not have any significant health complications and is not on any prescription medications. Whichever approach is selected, the individual seeking treatment should insure that the health professional chosen for treatment avails him/herself of others with the necessary expertise in dietary counseling, physical activity/exercise, and behavior modification/lifestyle changes as needed for success.

7.2.3 Diet

Dietary therapy consists in instructing patients on how to modify their diets and decrease caloric intake to achieve the desired target weight loss. Currently, it is recommended that most patients employ at least a moderate reduction in caloric intake and increase their physical activity/exercise to achieve a slow and progressive weight loss over time averaging 1-2 pounds a week.

The centerpiece of dietary therapy is a caloric restricted, low to moderate fat diet (LCD). It should contain nutrient composition that reduces risk factors such as elevated blood cholesterol, etc., as needed.

LCDs, along with physical activity/exercise, have been shown to reduce total body weight by 10-15% over a 6-month period of time. This is usually accompanied by a decease in waist circumference and waist to hip ratio. Weight lost in this manner usually consists principally of fat, and some muscle mass.

Dietary counseling/education is necessary in order to achieve adjustment to any LCD. Particular attention needs to be paid to the following:
*   alcohol consumption—limited or eliminated
*   avoiding over consumption of high calorie (high fat or high carbohydrate) foods
*   energy (caloric) content of different foods
*   food composition (fats, carbohydrates, protein, fiber, etc)
*   food preparation (reduce/avoid fats during cooking)
*   maintaining adequate water intake
*   establishing new purchasing habits—e.g., buying low calorie foods
*   reading nutrition labels for food composition and caloric content
*   reducing portion sizes

An average typical LCD may contain:

Calories	1200-1500 calories (1)
Total fat	25-30% of total calories (2)
Saturated fat	up to 10% of total calories
Monosaturated fat	up to 10% of total calories
Polyunsaturated fat	up to 10% of total calories
Cholesterol	300 mg/day
Protein	15% of total calories (3)
Carbohydrate	55% of total calories (4)
Calcium	1000-1500 mgm/day
Fiber	20-30 grams/day (5)
Vitamins/Minerals	as needed

1) adjusted to achieve 1-2 pound per week weight loss
2) patients with high blood cholesterol levels may need to further lower the amount and types of fat in the diet
3) protein should be derived from lean meat or fish or plant sources
4) mainly complex carbohydrates from different vegetables, fruits, and whole grains.
5) diets rich in soluble fiber, including oat bran, vegetables, barley, and most fruits may help reduce blood cholesterol levels, and aid in weight management by promoting satiety

Incorporating extra physical activity/exercise to expend an additional 300 or more calories a day, enables one to lose principally fat and reduce lean muscle mass loss.

Greater weight loss may be achieved by increasing the daily caloric deficit and/or increasing exercise accordingly. However, one must bear in mind that losing fat at a rate over 1-2 pounds per week may cause the body to reset the BMR lower so as to defend itself against "starvation". Therefore, it is important to increase exercise to keep the BMR at more "normal" levels so that when one achieves desired weight loss, weight will not easily be regained.

Caloric restriction involved in weight loss programs varies widely depending on the patient's degree of overweight or obesity and associated health risks/complications. A low calorie diet (LCD) generally is considered to be suitable and safe for most overweight/obese patients who:

• are attempting weight loss for the first time
• may have failed on one attempt to lose weight, but are reasonably well-motivated to lose weight and do not have major health risks/complications
• have a BMI less than 40

It should be remembered that diets prescribed and implemented by a dietician/nutritionist in a well-structured and supervised weight loss program are more likely to succeed, especially when it is the patient's first attempt at weight loss.

Basic nutritional proportions of ingredients in any diet should be consistent with Dietary Guidelines for Americans outlined by the US Department of Agriculture. Fluid intake should be at least 1.5 to 2.0 quarts of water daily unless chronic congestive heart failure, edema, kidney disease or some other clinical condition warrants otherwise.

Caloric intake and energy expenditure both need to be individualized to produce continued weight loss of approximately 1-2 pounds per week after the first month. Both need to be evaluated periodically (e.g., bimonthly by a dietician/healthcare professional, and/or physician) to help insure compliance and success.

Food logs/record books need to be completed regularly (e.g., weekly) by the patient to ensure adherence to dietary plan used.

Vitamin and mineral intake need to be adjusted according to the degree of caloric restriction and diet employed. Failure to do so may lead to deficiencies.

LCDs may be regarded as well-tolerated, safe and effective for most patients when prescribed and monitored by a health professional (e.g., dietician). However, some patients may develop complications that may require physician intervention. These may include such things as:
- dehydration
- excessive loss of lean body muscle mass
- cardiac arrhythmias
- vitamin and/or mineral deficiencies

If a patient needs to lose more than 1-2 pounds per week because of the degree of obesity and/or complications present, then additional caloric restriction or a very low caloric diet (VLCD) may be used under a physician's supervision.

VLCDs generally are not recommended for weight loss, except under special physician supervised circumstances, because:

- deficits are great and nutritional deficiencies will occur unless vitamin and mineral supplementation is added to the diet
- LCDs appear to be just as effective in producing weight loss in the long term
- while more weight is initially lost with VLCDs, more is usually regained afterwards
- patients using VLCDs are at increased risk for developing gallstones and other complications
- successful weight reduction is more likely to occur when consideration is given to a patient's food preferences, the LCD is tailored to an individual's needs, and all recommended dietary allowances are met.

VLCDs need to be individualized to patient needs. Such diets generally are considered appropriate when it is determined that:

- VLCD can be used safely
- a health risk/complication does not contradict use and the patient has a BMI of 30 or greater
- patient has failed in prior weight loss attempts in LCDs
- patient demonstrates necessary motivation to adhere to VLCD and necessary lifestyle change program to maintain weight loss
- patient is less than 65 years of age.

Generally, significantly more side effects and health risks are involved in the use of VLCDs compared to LCDs, especially if used by the patient alone without physician prescription and supervision. Drugs that may be required to treat complications of type 2 diabetes mellitus or hypertension, etc. may need to be reduced or discontinued to avoid side effects in patients on VLCDs. Other problems/side effects associated with VLCD use may include:

- gallstones in up to 25-30% of patients, especially in those with rapid or excessive weight loss
- excessive lean body muscle mass loss
- sudden death

Contraindications to use of VLCDs may include:

- recent heart attack (myocardial infarction)
- cardiac arrythmia/conduction defect
- type 1 diabetes mellitus (insulin dependent)
- gallbladder disease
- history of liver, kidney, or cerebrovascular disease
- AIDS

Patients who are on a VLCD usually require regular close medical supervision. Indiscriminate use of VLCDs by a patient without prescription/supervision by a physician is not recommended.

Generally the duration of VLCD therapy should not exceed 16 weeks in most patients. Longer use may lead to serious side effects such as excessive lean body muscle mass/nitrogen loss, gallstones, and ultimate relapse because transition to a more regular diet at the end of therapy can be psychologically and biologically difficult to achieve without significant weight gain and demotivation.

VLCDs usually produce at least 2 to 3 times more weight loss compared with LCDs, averaging around 3 or more pounds per week in women and 4 or more pounds per week in men. However, it should be noted that success in terms of weight loss achieved and maintained on VLCDs does not appear to be materially better than LCDs in most cases over the long term.

Dieting requires a good deal of planning for success. In planning any diet, Global Health and Fitness (http://www.global-fitness.com/foods/?partner=ghf) can provide you with the calorie, fat, carbohydrate, protein, fiber, sugar, cholesterol, sodium and alcohol content for thousands of foods, including fast foods prepared by over 100 popular restaurants.

Patient education materials for diets are available from the National Heart, Lung, and Blood Institute at:
http://www.nhbli.nih.gov/health/public/heart/obesity/lose_wt/shopping.htm
http://www.nhbli.nih.gov/health/public/heart/obesity/lose_wt/ob_tips.htm

For additional information, consult:
Cyberdiet
http://www.cyberdiet.com

FDA Center for Food Safety and Applied Nutrition
http://www.cfsan.fda.gov

USDA Center for Nutrition Policy Promotion
http://www.usda.gov/cnpp

USDA Nutrient Data Laboratory
http://www.nal.usda.fnic/foodcomp

7.2.4 Physical Activity/Exercise

- **Introduction**

Physical activity in primary prevention of overweight and obesity ideally should begin in the early school years of a child and continue through an individual's lifetime.

Walking generally is the recommended mode of physical activity/exercise for most individuals.

Moderate physical activity/exercise alone produces only a modest amount of weight loss over the long term in most patients. Significant weight loss usually can only be achieved using a combination of caloric restriction and regular, moderate-intensity daily physical activity/exercise.

A progressive decrease in the amount of energy expended for work, transportation, and personal activities is believed by many to be a major factor in overweight and obesity in the US and the Western world. Therefore, a moderate-intensity daily physical activity/exercise program is considered essential for weight loss.

- **Benefits**

In combination with caloric restriction, moderate-intensity daily physical activity/exercise:
- burns calories and increases the caloric deficit and weight loss
- improves lean body mass, and minimizes muscle loss
- improves cardiovascular and general fitness and the risk of complications
- decreases insulin resistance and type 2 diabetes mellitus
- reduces blood cholesterol, body fat and the risk of cardiovascular disease

- reduces feelings of anxiety, depression and stress, and elevates sense of well-being
- improves fitness, mobility and the ability to perform activities of daily living

One should bear in mind that many of the benefits of physical activity/exercise occur even if one remains overweight or obese. There is a significantly lower mortality rate in the physically active compared to those who remain sedentary.

- **Examples for Consideration**

Most professionals in the field have recommended at least 30-60 minutes of moderate-intensity physical activity/exercise 5-7 times a week, however, the Institute of Medicine now recommends at least 1 hour per day. Whether the adopted program is 30-60 minutes or longer, exercise confers substantial benefits in itself, so that if one is unable to move up to 1 hour or longer daily exercise level, then the 30 minute standard may suffice.

To be successful, a physical activity/exercise program needs to be done at a comfort level and easily fit into an individual's daily living routine/schedule on a regular basis, 5-7 days a week. One should start out slowly and gradually increase activity/exercise to moderate-intensity over the course of a few weeks time. Trying too hard at first may lead to injury and prove to be counterproductive.

Examples of moderate-intensity physical activity/exercise include:

Common Activities

- washing and waxing the car for 45-60 minutes
- washing windows or floors for 45-60 minutes

- gardening for 30-45 minutes
- raking leaves for 30-45 minutes
- walking 2 miles in 30 minutes (15 minute mile)
- shoveling snow for 30-40 minutes
- stair climbing for 20-25 minutes

Sporting Activities/Exercises

- playing volleyball for 30-45 minutes
- playing touch football for 30-45 minutes
- shooting basketballs for 30-45 minutes
- bicycling 5 miles in 30 minutes
- dancing fast (social) for 30 minutes
- water aerobics for 30 minutes
- swimming freestyle for 30 minutes
- playing a basket ball game for 20 minutes

Gym/Home Activities

- exercise video for 60 minutes
- walking/jogging on a treadmill for 45-60 minutes
- using a stairmaster machine for 25-30 minutes
- lifting weights/using body building equipment for 30-40 minutes
- jumping rope for 20 minutes

Other opportunities for increasing physical activity include:
- using the stairs instead of the elevator
- parking at a significant distance from the mall/store/theater and walking to the door and back to the car
- taking a 5-10 minute walk before or after meals
- cleaning the house
- mowing the lawn

An exercise program can be done all at one time, or divided into segments over the course of each day. Walking is a particularly attractive form of physical activity/exercise because of its benefits, relative safety, easy accessibility and very low cost. One can start out walking slowly for 15-30 minutes, 1-2 days a week and gradually build up to 60 minutes or more of moderate–intensity brisk walking 5-7 days a week. The goal is to burn an extra 300 or more calories per day, or 1500-2000 calories per week, with exercise.

Bear in mind that estimates of calories burned per activity is not an exact science—merely a rough estimate at best. Heavier and/or younger persons and males tend to burn more calories per activity than females. Exercising harder and faster increases calories burned however, it is better to exercise for a longer time rather than harder and faster. Figures provided are considered as useful estimates by which to help balance daily caloric expenditure versus intake for weight maintenance, or to calculate desired caloric deficit for weight loss diets.

To obtain an estimate of calories you may burn performing different activities/exercises, consult: http://www.caloriesperhour.com. This Web site provide you with:
- calories burned per activity
- your body mass index (BMI) calculator
- your basal metabolic rate (BMR) calculator

Once on this Web site:
- select an activity/exercise
- enter time in hours and/or minutes
- enter your weight in pounds, height in feet and inches, sex and age
- press "calculate" for "calorie burn", BMI and BMR estimates

Note you can enter a number of activities you plan to perform daily to obtain total "calorie burn" per day. For example, for a 250 pound, 5'10" male, age 30, "calorie burn" for the following activities is estimated as:

- back packing, hilly, 30 minutes   340 calories
- ballroom dancing, fast, 30 minutes   375 calories
- bicycling, flat surface, moderate, 30 minutes   330 calories
- bike, stationary, 30 minutes   330 calories
- cleaning/waxing car, 45 minutes   325 calories
- cleaning house, moderate, 60 minutes   300 calories
- disco dancing, fast, 40 minutes   330 calories
- handball, singles, 20 minutes   350+ calories
- hiking, 10 lb. load, hilly, 30 minutes   330 calories
- jogging in place, 30 minutes   350+ calories
- raking leaves, moderate, 45 minutes   310 calories
- rope jumping, moderate, 20 minutes   320 calories
- rowing, stationary, moderate, 30 minutes   340 calories
- snow shoveling, 40 minutes   350+ calories
- stair climbing, 20-25 minutes   350+ calories
- swimming, freestyle, 30 minutes   330 calories
- tennis, singles, 30 minutes   350+ calories
- touch football (beach), 30 minutes   350+ calories
- walking (3.5 mph) on level, 60 minutes   350+ calories
- walking (3.0 mph) uphill, 60 minutes   350+ calories
- working out at gym, 30 minutes   320 calories

Click on questions and obtain answers to help you learn basics of diet, exercise, and weight loss.

For additional information, consult Global Health and Fitness at: http://www.global-fitness.com

- **Walking for Weight Loss/Fitness/Health**

A walking program may include activities designed for:
- weight loss—moderate-intensity walking helps flatten the stomach muscles, reduce hips, tone thighs and leg muscles, decrease excess body fat and aid weight loss.
- cardiovascular conditioning—higher intensity walking helps strengthen the heart muscles, improves aerobic endurance, enables one to perform better in aerobic activities, and recover more quickly from physical exertion
- muscle toning—combines walking with more special resistance training to increase muscle mass, and improve muscle endurance, body firmness, and resting metabolism
- long term health—for the dedicated walker seeking long term health, increased energy, reduced stress and fatigue, and a reduction in the risk of cardiovascular disease, and type 2 diabetes mellitus, etc. as well as improved mood and self esteem and an increase in longevity.

Walking for weight loss requires a combination of an appropriate walking/exercise program and dietary, caloric and fat restriction. Walking at a moderate-intensity 5-7 days a week is generally regarded as an effective way to lose weight and become reasonably fit. To implement such a program, one needs to determine a walking target heart rate pace that can be maintained for 60 minutes or longer without undue fatigue, shortness of breath, or muscle tightness/soreness.

- **Target Heart Rate/Weight Loss**

Typically, a reasonable walking pace for target weight loss tends to be around 3-4 miles per hour for 60 minutes, 5-7 times a week. Less intensive or less frequent walking programs generally tend not to be as effective.

Generally, the longer and more often one walks, the more calories/fat will be burnt, and the more weight lost.

One can estimate their walking target heart rate for weight loss by using the Karvonen formula as below:

(220–A–RHR) x 50–60%+RHR=THR (where A=age in years, RHR=resting heart rate and THR=target heart rate).

220–A (age in years)=predicted maximum heart rate (MHR)

MHR–RHR (resting heart rate)=HRR (heart rate reserve)

Multiplying the HRR by 50–60% plus the RHR sets the upper and lower THR limits in beats per minute

RHR is determined by taking your pulse for one minute before arising out of bed in the morning for 3 consecutive days and averaging the results

Thus, if one is 30 years old with RHR of 70, weight loss THR will be 130 at the 50% level and 142 at the 60% level.

One who is 55 years old with RHR of 65 would have a THR of 115 at the 50% level and 125 at the 60% level

A Global Health and Fitness "Heart Rate Calculator" based on the Karvonen Formula and exercise guidelines from the American College of Sports Medicine can be found at:
http://www.global-fitness.com/heartcalc_intro.html

Once determined, an individual needs to start walking/exercising at a comfortable heart rate below the lower level THR and gradually, over the course of the first couple of weeks, work up to an effective, well-tolerated and safe THR within limits and walk continuously at that level for 60 minutes 5-7 days a week. If time is a problem for the 60 minute walk, then three separate 20 minute walks, or two 30 minute walks daily at the THR should produce essentially the same results. Therefore, one should not become discouraged if a continuous 60-minute THR walk cannot be done. Walking can be done outdoors weather permitting, or in a mall, at home, in a gym, or on a treadmill.

Followed consistently over time, such a THR walking program should allow one to log 17-24 miles per week for a total weekly caloric expenditure of around 1500-2100 calories. As a pound of body fat is equivalent to around 3500 calories, one may burn around 0.4 to 0.6 pounds of excess fat weekly in this way, or 21-31 pounds per year from walking alone. Coupling such a THR walking weight loss program with other physical activities and caloric restriction of at least 500-1000 calories per day, weight loss of 1-2 pounds per week may be produced.

• **Target Heart Rate/Cardiovascular Conditioning/Fitness**

For cardiovascular conditioning/fitness, one needs to focus more on intensity rather than duration of walking. Heart and lungs need to be worked hard enough to produce a significant conditioning (training) effect, and this involves a "sweat-producing" walking pace reaching a THR of around 70 to 80% of MHR. To find your THR for cardiovascular conditioning/fitness, substitute 70-80% in place of 50-60% in the previous equation. Thus, for example, for someone 30 years of age with a resting heart rate of 70, cardiovascular conditioning/fitness THR is calculated to be 154 beats per minute at the 70% level and 166 beats per minute at the 80% level.

Cardiovascular condition/fitness requires walking at this 70-80% of maximum heart rate for at least 20-30 minutes or more 3-4 times per week. It should be noted that such a walking/exercise program is shorter in duration and more intense than that required for just weight loss. Such a 20-30 minute brisk, continuous walking program plus a brief "warm up" before, and "cool down" afterwards done every other day at a cardiovascular conditioning/fitness THR weekly may be sufficient. Bear in mind that a brisk walking program means walking between 3.75 mph (16 minute mile) and 4.3 mph (14 minute mile) averaging 4 mph. And, walking at around 4 miles per hour for 30 minutes means burning 350-400 or more calories of energy.

Incorporating some basic race walking techniques usually helps one reach cardiovascular conditioning/fitness pace more easily. Such techniques include bending your arms to a 90-degree angle, swinging them like a pendulum at your side while you walk, and taking short steps as quickly as possible.

It should be noted that the Karvonen formula for estimating THR is considered to be applicable and useful for most overweight and obese individuals providing they do not have significant other health complications. However, it needs to be recognized that this formula has limited application in patients with cardiovascular and other diseases as adverse symptoms may occur before THR can be achieved. Thus, in patients with heart disease, for example, a treadmill exercise test by a physician, may be considered more appropriate to determine safe limits of physical activity/exercise/walking.

• **Muscle Mass/Toning**

Muscle mass and toning are essential for maintaining basal metabolic rate, fitness and ability to burn calories and fat. Remember that muscle "burns calories", fat more or less just "sits there"—and fat bodies perform rather poorly in terms of "fuel burning". Toned muscle mass enables one to more effectively burn calories, support weight, work more effectively, play at sports, perform well under stress, lift more weight, and help to compensate for any loss of bone that may occur as one ages.

Walking even at low speeds and heart rates improves leg muscle mass and tone. However, to more effectively build muscle mass and increase tone, one needs to walk/exercise against resistance. And, gravity is the easiest resistance for a walker to use. Simply walking up anything—hills, stairs, inclined treadmill, stair climbing, etc., will work leg muscles to advantage against resistance and help build muscle mass and increase muscle tone—principally in the legs.

On the other hand, toning the upper body while walking involves using such things as hand–held weights or weight resistance bands. Light hand or wrist weight bands increase the upper body workload building muscle mass/tone in the arms, shoulders, and chest, especially when one swings the arms close to the body while walking. Using a stretch band loop around the handrails while walking on a treadmill and pumping the arms in a mutual walking rhythm against the stretching resistance of the band helps increase upper body muscle mass/tone. Lifting weights/using body building equipment in a gym or at home is another way to build muscle mass/tone.

• **Long Term Health**

Long-term health benefits may be achieved by "life-long" walking. Only five to seven weekly 300-calorie daily walks/workouts should help get you there—each 60 minutes of moderate-intensity 3-4 miles per hour walking. Health improvement gains above the 2000 calories a week "burn" rate are only marginally better.

Six relatively easy walking ways to burn 300 calories or more per day include:
- 60 minutes of level moderate-paced walking
- 30-45 minutes of level brisk-paced walking
- 30-45 minutes of hill-trail or inclined treadmill walking
- 30-45 minutes of fast ballroom dancing
- 20-25 minutes of stairmaster climbing
- 30 minutes of hilly hiking with 10 lb. back pack load at 3.0 mph

Remember, if cardiovascular conditioning is not one of your goals, then walking speed and intensity can be lowered. Once desired weight is lost, and further weight loss is no longer of major concern, longer distances and intensity can be de-emphasized accordingly while continuing the walking/exercise program.

- **Achieve Better Walking Skills**

To achieve better walking skills, one should adopt:
- relaxed movements for fast, efficient walking
- good posture keeping the lower back flat and abdominal muscles contracted putting the pelvis into healthy alignment with the spinal column eliminating any sway back or lumbar lordosis
- controlled abdominal exercises between walks
- using arms bent at a 90 degree angle and letting them swing like a pendulum while walking—remembering that a short pendulum swings faster. Arms and legs should move in synchrony—faster arm swings, quicker steps

- short quick steps to accelerate walking speed—not longer ones remembering that a 4 miles per hour pace is around 130 steps or more per minute on average
- avoid sore shins by gradually increasing speed of walking to get shin muscles in shape. Use walking shoes instead of thick-heeled running shoes to avoid sore shins. Shin muscles pull the toes up when the heel strikes the ground, and the faster one walks, the higher the toes are at heel-strike
- practical rules include:
  - walk fast enough to notice breathing without becoming out of breath
  - pause to breathe as necessary while having a conversation with a walking partner
  - sweat mildly to moderately as elevated body temperature accompanies harder work involved in burning more calories
  - rest afterwards for muscle tissue rebuilding

Finally, whenever possible, it is prudent for anyone who is overweight or obese, with or without health complications, to consult a physician before embarking on any exercise program. Consultation with an exercise physiologist may also be helpful.

For additional information, consult:
U.S. Department of Health and Human Services
Report on: *Physical Activity Fundamental to Preventing Disease*
http:// aspe.hhs.gov/health/reports/physicalactivity

National Heart, Lung and Blood Institute
Report on: *Guide to Physical Activity*
http://www.nhlbi.nih.gov/health/public/heart/obesity/lose_wt/phy_act
.htm

Report on: *Guidelines on Overweight and Obesity: Electronic Textbook: Physical Activity*
http://www.nhlbi.nih.gov/guidelines/obesity/e_txtbk/txgd/4322.htm

Just Move.Org
Report on: *How to Implement Physical Activity in Primary and Secondary Prevention*
http://www.justmove.org

Shape Up America
http://www.shapeup.org

7.2.5 Behavior Modification/Counseling/Education

Behavior modification/counseling/education strategies are used to help one achieve desired target weight loss. Unless one acquires a new and more appropriate behavior including a new set of eating and physical activity habits, long term weight reduction and maintenance is not likely to succeed. As a result, patients, healthcare staff, and physicians need to become familiar with behavior modification techniques/strategies and use them for modifying behavior accordingly.

Behavior modification strategies provide methods for overcoming barriers to compliance with needed changes. Education about nutrition, diet, and physical activity/exercise is very important. Strategies need to be individualized for each patient.

No single behavior modification strategy/technique or combination of behavioral methods has been found to be superior. Behavioral change can be achieved either on an individual basis or in group settings. The group approach has the advantages of lower cost and group support, and appears to be more successful for most individuals.

Behavioral strategies may include:

- cognitive restructuring

  Unrealistic goals and beliefs about weight loss and body image and self-defeating thoughts and feelings that undermine weight loss efforts need to be modified

- contingency management

  Verbal and tangible rewards are used to decrease sedentary time spent, increase time spent walking and exercising, reduce consumption of unhealthy foods and decrease caloric intake.

- problem solving

  Setbacks are re-evaluated. Individuals are helped to learn from their mistakes rather than punish themselves with negative thoughts, feelings, and behavior. Brainstorming solutions to impediments to weight loss, and planning and implementing healthier alternatives are techniques employed.

- self-monitoring

  Recording of daily activities, eating habits and comments is a key to behavior modification. Patients are instructed on how to record the amount and types of physical activity, food eaten, caloric values, and nutrient composition in order for the patient to gain insight to personal behavior. Recording of feelings/comments regarding behavior serves to bring previously unrecognized unhealthful habits to light for correction.

- stress management

  Stress commonly triggers dysfunctional eating patterns/overeating and failure to exercise properly. Management techniques are used to defuse stressful situations leading to overeating. Coping strategies used include meditation and relaxation techniques, etc.

- stimulus control

  Patients are educated to shop carefully for healthy foods, and to avoid purchasing unhealthy ones, keep high calorie foods out of

the house, limit times and places for eating, and avoid situations in which overeating occurs.
- social support
  Social support from family, friends, colleagues and a support group are used to facilitate weight reduction and maintenance, and provide positive reinforcement. Parents and children are encouraged to work together and engage in and maintain healthy dietary and physical activity habits.

Patients suffering from binge eating disorder may need to be referred to a health professional who specializes in that field.

For additional information, consult:

National Heart, Lung and Blood Institute
- Report on: *Guide to Behavior Change*
  http://www.nhlbi.nih.gov/health/public/heart/obesity/lose_wt/behavior.htm

7.2.6 Weight Reduction in the Elderly

Whether weight reduction leads to significantly increased survival among the elderly (>age 65) remains to be demonstrated in well–controlled clinical trials.

The importance of treating overweight/obesity at older ages has been questioned because:
- epidemiological studies suggest a decreased significance of relative risk at older ages
- potential adverse effects of treatment have been raised with respect to dietary deficiencies and bone loss increasing the risk of fractures from weight loss regimens

- involuntary weight loss indicative of occult disease such as cancer may easily be mistaken for success in voluntary weight loss in a weight management program

In spite of all this, most experts in the field still believe that age alone should not preclude treatment of overweight/obesity elderly men and women. Therefore, a clinical decision, not to undertake treatment in an older adult should be guided by an evaluation of potential benefits regarding:

- day-to-day functioning
- reduction of future cardiovascular, and other complications
- individual's motivation for weight reduction
- likelihood of preventing adverse effects on bone and nutritional deficiencies

For additional information, consult:

National Heart, Lung and Blood Institute
Report on: *Guidelines on Overweight and Obesity: Electronic Textbook: Weight Reduction After Age 65*
http://www.nhbli.nih.gov/guidelines/obesity/e_txtbk/txgd/452.htm

7.3   Drugs/Pharmacotherapy

7.3.1 Overview

Overweight/obesity is a chronic disease that requires long term treatment. As in other chronic diseases, use of prescription drugs may be considered appropriate in some patients. Drug therapy with prescription medications is referred to as pharmacotherpay and drugs used are called either anti-obesity or anorectic agents. Ordinarily, drugs are not recommended in the treatment of overweight patients without complications who are not considered to be obese—those with a BMI of 25.0-29.9 –because weight loss and maintenance thereof in such individuals usually can be achieved without the use of drugs.

Anti-obesity/anorectic prescription medications should be used only under the direct supervision of a physician. They should be:
- approved by the Food and Drug Administration
- used as adjuncts to lifestyle changes, diet, exercise and behavior modification
- employed generally for no more than 1 year—possibly up to 2 years in selected patients
- considered appropriate and suitable for select obese patients with a BMI of 30 or greater with no health complications, and with a BMI 27.0-29.9 and at least one major complication (e.g., type 2 diabetes mellitus, cardiovascular disease, etc.)

Some obese patients prescribed pharmacotherapy and supervised by a physician may be more likely to achieve desired target weight loss and maintenance. However, it needs to be recognized that around 30% or more of obese patients fail to respond satisfactorily to anti-obesity/anorectic agents. Also, such drugs are only modestly effective in most patients. Nevertheless, if weight loss of 10-15% or greater is achieved after 6 months or so of treatment, and weight loss is continuing, pharmacotherapy may be continued at the doctor's discretion if the patient fully appreciates the risk/benefits involved. Realistically, however, total weight loss greater than 10-15% of initial body weight is the exception and not the rule. Most patients that lose more than 15% of initial body weight usually do so without the use of prescription drugs.

There is some clinical evidence that anti-obesity/anorectic drugs may be useful in the long-term maintenance of weight loss in some patients. However, the evidence is neither substantial or very convincing and the long term efficacy and safety remains to be established in large-scale, well-controlled clinical trials beyond 1 year.

Most studies of anti-obesity/anorectic drugs indicate that weight loss tends to level off after 6-12 months of therapy, even though the patient is still on medication. While some patients and physicians may be concerned that this may indicate tolerance to the mediation, leveling off of weight may mean that the medication has reached its level of effectiveness, and weight gain may ensue.

7.3.2 FDA Approved Anti-obesity/Anoretic Agents

US Food and Drug Administration approved anti-obesity agents include:

	Generic Name	DEA Schedule	Mode of Action	Use
1.	Benzphetamine (Didrex)	III	S/AS	ST
2.	Phendimetrozine (Bontril)	III	S/AS	ST
3.	Phentermine (Adipex-P)	IV	S/AS	ST
4.	Phentermine Resin SR* (Ionamin)	IV	S/AS	ST
5.	Diethylpropion (Tenuate)	IV	S/AS	ST
6.	Sibutramine (Meridia)	IV	S/AS	LT
7.	Orlistate (Xenical)	not required	gut lipase inhibitor	LT

TM=trade mark name for each drug is given in parentheses below the generic name

*SR=sustained release form of drug

DEA=Drug Enforcement Agency Schedule. Numbers indicate degree of abuse/addiction potential. Schedule I drugs have the greatest and Schedule IV the least abuse/addiction potential. A drug not requiring scheduling by the DEA is regarded as having no significant abuse/addiction potential.

S=stimulant (e.g., central nervous system)

AS=appetite suppressant (anorectic agent)

ST=short term, few weeks to a few months

LT=long term, up to 1 year or possibly more in select cases

7.3.3 Anti-obesity/Anorectic Drug Use/Results

The FDA has approved most stimulant anorectic agents for short-term use—meaning weeks to months. Sibutramine and orlistat are the only drugs approved for use up to 1 year. Use of these drugs for longer than 1 year remains to be established in well-controlled clinical trials. However, a physician has the right to prescribe such drugs for a greater length of time as an "off label" use under the law in select patients keeping in mind that only a few well-controlled clinical trials of more than 2 years in duration that have evaluated the safety and effectiveness of these agents.

Combinations of anti-obesity/anorectic agents is "off label" and experimental in nature, and should be entertained only with caution under special circumstances, if at all. Combined treatment with fenfluramine and phentermine ("fen/phen") is no longer available due to withdrawal of the combination from the marketplace because of toxicity. Little information is available regarding the safety and effectiveness of other drug combinations and such also remains "off label" and experimental at this time.

Most of the available drugs are classified as appetite suppressants (anorectic agents) as they generally are believed to promote weight loss by decreasing appetite and/or increasing the feeling of being full. Such effects are considered to be related to levels of brain catecholamines and/or serotonin, brain chemicals that affect mood and appetite. In contrast, orlistat works by reducing the body's ability to absorb dietary fat from the gut by approximately one third by inhibiting the enzyme lipase that breaks down fat in the gut for absorption.

Approved anti-obesity/anorectic agents are generally considered to be well-tolerated and safe for short-term use in most patients. However, one needs to bear in mind that:
- these drugs should not be used for cosmetic purposes just to improve appearance
- significant side effects may occur and such drugs should be used selectively and carefully
- prescription weight loss drugs generally are used if there is inability to lose weight or maintain weight loss on basic medical treatment
- certain other concomitant medical disorders or medication being taken by an individual may negatively influence a physician's decision to prescribe weight loss drugs
- they should not be used to replace lifestyle changes, caloric restriction, physical activity, and behavior modification
- obesity is a chronic disease and treatment needs to be continued for years, and long-term safety and efficacy are not yet established
- most individuals who stop taking weight-loss drugs usually regain a significant amount, if not all, weight lost
- there is no one recommended drug or dose for all patients. A physician needs to decide which drug and dose may be appropriate, effective, and safe for a given individual.

While side effects generally are mild to moderate in nature and usually diminish in intensity with continued treatment, serious, and rarely even fatal outcomes, have been reported. Among the more serious side effects are drug abuse/addiction and cardiovascular and other toxicity.

Drug abuse/addiction is an ever present potential danger with all DEA scheduled drugs. Benzphetamine and phendimetrazine, DEA Schedule III agents, appear to have the greatest potential for abuse/addiction. Phentermine, phentermine resin, diethylpropion, and sibutramine are DEA Schedule IV drugs. They are considered less likely to produce abuse or addiction, however, some risk for this is still present. However, abuse/addiction is not commonly encountered in patients who are carefully counseled and supervised by their prescribing physician.

Stimulant appetite suppressant agents are prone to produce significant central nervous system stimulation and/or cardiovascular side effects. Patients may develop nervousness, euphoria, difficulty in sleeping, or elevation of blood pressure and/or pulse, etc. Serious cardiovascular toxicity has been reported to have occurred with the combination of fenfluramine and phentermine ("fen/phen"), and fenfluramine plus dexfenfluramine ("fen/dex"), and these combinations had to be withdrawn from the market. A few reports of cardiovascular toxicity (e.g., primary pulmonary hypertension) also have been reported with the use of phentermine alone.

Thus, long term use of stimulant appetite suppressants alone or in combination cannot be recommended until safety and efficacy can be demonstrated in large-scale, well-controlled clinical trials, substantial enough to permit FDA approval of such use.

Sibutramine and orlistat are the only medications approved for longer-term use in obese patients.

Sibutramine (Meridia) is a central nervous system stimulant anorectic agent that reduces food intake and may even increase energy (caloric) expenditure. When used in combination with basic medical treatment, sibutramine is regarded as effective for weight loss and maintenance for up to 1 year. Weight loss of at least 4 pounds in the first 4 weeks of treatment with the drug is correlated with significant further weight loss, reduction in body mass index, decrease in waist-to-hip ratio and waist circumference as well as blood cholesterol and triglycerides in most patients. Sibutramine generally is regarded as well-tolerated, effective, and safe, and having a low abuse/addiction potential.

Orlistat (Xenical) is an anti-obesity agent with a novel mode of action. It binds, and inactivates, pancreatic lipase (which is involved in the absorption of fat) in the intestinal tract decreasing dietary fat absorption into the body. Clinical trials indicate that orlistat may produce significantly more weight loss compared with placebo in over half of the patients over the course of treatment for 1 year. Because the drug can interfere with the absorption of fat-soluble vitamins, particularly D and E, supplementation of diet with fat-soluble vitamins is needed. Multivitamin tablets should be taken 2 hours before or after orlistat to minimize interference with the absorption of fat-soluble vitamins. The drug generally is regarded as reasonably well-tolerated, efficacious, and safe for treatment for up to one year.

Benzphetamine, phendimetrazine, phentermine, phentermine resin, and diethylpropion are stimulant anorectic agents approved for short-term use, a few weeks to months, treatment. Patients taking these drugs may lose up to 25 pounds or so over a 6 month or so period of time. While they generally are regarded as reasonably well-tolerated, efficacious, and safe in most, a significant number of patients may not be able to complete a prescribed course of short term therapy because of side effects and/or lack of efficacy, and discontinue drug treatment as a result.

Over-the-counter (OTC) dietary supplements/herbs/drugs, used to lose weight, are not regarded as sufficiently efficacious and safe to be recommended. Phenylpropanolamine, ephedrine, and Ma Huang, (containing ephedrine), are not very efficacious and appear to be widely abused. They may produce powerful stimulant effects on the heart and central nervous system with undesirable consequences.

For additional information, consult:

National Institute of Diabetes and Digestive and Kidney Disease
• Report on: *Prescription Mediations for the Treatment of Obesity*
  http://www.niddk.nih.gov/health/nutrit/pubs/presmeds.htm

American Academy of Family Practice
• Report on: *Drug Therapy for Obesity*
  http://www.aafp.org/afp/20000615/3615.html

US Food and Drug Administration
http://www.fda.gov (search "prescription anti-obesity drugs")

Drug Info Net
http://www.druginfonet.com (search "weight loss drugs")

National Center for Complimentary and Alternative Medicine
http://www.nccam.nih.gov

7.4   Surgical Treatment

7.4.1 Overview

Severe obesity is a chronic disease with substantial health and economic consequences, and is very difficult to treat medically successfully.

Therefore, surgery, to promote weight loss by restricting food/caloric intake and interrupting digestive absorption/ processes, is becoming an increasingly used option.

It is estimated that around 70,000-80,000 of 10-15 million or more severely obese Americans now have been treated surgically, and this figure is expected to grow rapidly in coming years as techniques improve and more is known about the long term results.

Currently, surgical intervention may be considered for carefully selected patients who are:
- between 18 and 65 years of age
- severely obese for at least 5 years or more, and have failed to achieve satisfactory weight loss on basic medical treatment and drugs
- not suffering from a significant psychiatric or psychological disorder
- at least 100 pounds overweight and have a BMI of 40 or greater, or a BMI of 35-39.9 along with one or more life threatening or disabling complications such as uncontrolled type 2 diabetes mellitus, essential hypertension, or cardiopulmonary disease such as sleep apnea
- considered to be highly motivated and able to accept and carry out necessary lifestyle, diet, exercise, and behavior modification changes required for success

While surgery appears to produce significant sustained weight loss in severely obese patients, it is not without its risks. Both the perioperative and long-term complications, and risk/benefit ratio needs to be carefully evaluated in each case bearing in mind that life-long medical/surgical surveillance after surgery is required.

7.4.2 Surgical Options

• **Introduction**

Normally, as food is ingested and moves along the digestive tract, digestive juices and enzymes digest and enhance the absorption of food. After chewing, and swallowing, food moves down the esophagus to the stomach where gastric acid aids in the digestive process. The stomach normally holds around 3 pints of food at any one time. When the stomach completes its digestive processes, contents move on into the duodenum, the first segment of the small intestine, and bile from the gallbladder and enzymes from the pancreas, increase the digestive process and absorption of food calories and nutrients. Most of the iron and calcium in the foods we eat are absorbed in the duodenum. Remaining food, ingredients, and intestinal digestive juices move on to the next two segments of the small intestine, the jejunum and subsequently the ileum, where remaining food particles and nutrients are absorbed. Thus, in the approximately 20 feet of small intestine, almost all food calories and nutrients are absorbed. Those food particles that cannot be digested in the small intestine move on to the large intestine and are stored there until eliminated in the feces. Some food nutrients also may be eliminated in the urine, especially when ingested in excess

Surgical options used in the treatment of severe obesity are designed to restrict food/caloric intake or create malabsorption of food calories. This may be done in essentially two basic surgical ways, namely: 1) restriction procedures and 2) combination of restriction and malabsorption procedures

• **Restriction Procedures**

Restriction procedures are commonly employed. Food intake into the stomach is restricted by creating a small thumb-sized pouch, holding around 1 ounce of food initially, at the top of the stomach where food enters from the esophagus. Capacity of the pouch, may expand to 2-3 ounces over time as food is consumed. The pouch's lower outlet to the rest of the stomach is constructed to have a small diameter of around one half inch that serves to delay emptying into the remainder of the stomach, creating a feeling of fullness.

After such a restriction procedure, the patient usually can eat only around one half to a whole cup of food without feeling full, or creating stomach discomfort or nausea, thus limiting food/caloric intake accordingly. Also, food ingested has to be well-chewed in order to exit the pouch successfully. Therefore, for most people with this type of operation, the ability to eat a large amount of food at any one time is lost. However, some patients may be able to return to eating modest amounts of food over time as the pouch expands.

Restriction procedures employed for surgical treatment include: gastric banding (GB), laparoscopic adjustable gastric banding (LAGB), and vertical banded gastroplasty (VBG)).

Gastric banding (GB) uses a special plastic material surgically placed around the upper portion of the stomach creating a small pouch with a narrow passage into the larger remainder of the stomach. Clinical results with this procedure have not been very impressive and it has been largely replaced by other surgical procedures.

LAGB was approved by the US Food and Drug Administration for the treatment of severe obesity in June 2001. However, a number of university and other surgical centers still are not offering LAGB because weight loss results to date do not appear to be as good as with the Roux-En-Y Gastric Bypass (discussed later in this chapter).

LAGB involves laparoscopic implantation of an adjustable silicone band with a balloon at the end which can be inflated with saline from a port implanted under the skin of the abdomen producing a small gastric pouch (in the upper part of the stomach) with a small opening emptying into the remainder of the stomach. The ring (around the lower end of the pouch) produced by the inflated band controls the flow of food from the pouch to the rest of the stomach and digestive tract. Thus, the patient is made to feel full with a small amount of food. Because of the slow emptying of the pouch, the patient may continue to feel full for several hours after eating, and the urge to eat between meals is reduced.

One of the reported advantages of LAGB is that the stoma size (exit from the pouch to the remainder of the stomach) can be adjusted postoperatively on an outpatient basis to control the flow of food into the rest of the stomach and digestive tract. Also, as the laparoscopic procedure is less invasive than traditional open surgery, less surgical complications and faster recovery are reported to be the rule.

VBG traditionally had been one of the more commonly used restrictive surgical procedures for treating severe obesity. This procedure employed an implanted band and gastric staples to create a small pouch at the top of the stomach with a restricted opening to the rest of the stomach. Results unfortunately were not as "good" as originally reported and the procedure is no longer used widely today.

Restriction procedures generally lead to significant weight loss in almost all patients, averaging up to 40-50% of overweight. Around 30% of patients are reported to achieve normal weight over time. However, some patients remain unable to cope effectively with lifestyle, diet, exercise and either fail to achieve target weight loss or do not maintain weight loss.

Complications of restrictive procedures not uncommonly occur and may include:

- nausea/vomiting due to overstretching of the stomach pouch with food portions that are too large or not well chewed
- band slippage/erosions requiring corrective re-operation
- breakdown of gastric staple line with leakage of stomach juices into the peritoneal cavity requiring emergency surgical correction
- wound infection

Death is reported to occur in less than 0.5% of cases.

- **Roux-En-Y Gastric Bypass**

Roux-En-Y Gastric Bypass (REY-GP) procedure combines the creation of a small stomach pouch to restrict food/caloric intake with the construction of a bypass of the lower portion of the stomach and the duodenum into the lower portions of the small intestine to cause malabsorption of food/calories.

Because of encouraging results to date, the REY-GP procedure appears to be the most common surgical procedure done in most university centers for the treatment of severe obesity today.

In this procedure, a small pouch is created in the upper portion of the stomach via gastric stapling or vertical banding to restrict food intake. Then a Y-shaped section of the small intestine is fashioned surgically. One end is attached to the lower, exit end of the stomach pouch, and the other end to the lower portion of the small intestine allowing partially digested food to bypass the duodenum and the first part of the jejunum. This procedure reduces food/calorie/nutrient absorption from the small intestine resulting in malabsorption.

The REY-GB procedure is reported to produce more weight loss compared with purely restriction operations because it adds the malabsorption aspect to enhance the caloric deficit. Patients are reported to lose from two-thirds to three-quarters or more on average of their excess weight over normal within approximately two years postoperatively.

The procedure may be done by open surgery, or laparoscopically in certain centers skilled in this approach.

Return to full activity usually occurs within 8 weeks following open surgery and sooner following the procedure done laparoscopically.

Death is reported to occur in less than 0.5% of patients.

Because REY-GB causes food/nutrients to bypass the duodenum where most of the iron and calcium and other nutrients are absorbed, the risk for nutritional deficiencies is higher. Anemia also may result from malabsorption of vitamin B-12 and iron deficiency may occur particularly in menstruating women. Decreased absorption of calcium may result in osteopenia and/or osteoporosis. Patients given supplements of these nutrients usually can avoid such complications.

The gastric bypass aspect of the REY-GB procedure may also cause the "dumping syndrome". Stomach contents may move too rapidly through the stomach and small intestine producing nausea, weakness, sweating, and not uncommonly, diarrhea after eating. Also, eating sweets can cause the patient to become so weak and sweaty as to require lying down until the symptoms ameliorate.

The more extensive the gastric bypass produced, the greater the risk for complications and nutritional deficiencies. Patients with such extensive bypass operations require not only close monitoring but also life-long use of special foods and medication.

A more extensive gastric bypass operation called biliopancreatic diversion, involving removal of portions of the stomach and connecting the small gastric pouch directly to the final segment of the small intestine (ileum), completely bypasses the duodenum and jejunum. It is not widely used anymore because of the higher risk of complications and nutritional deficiencies.

7.4.3 Overall Surgical Results

With surgical intervention, most severely obese individuals lose weight rapidly, and continue to do so for at least 18-24 months after the procedure. Some patients may then start to regain a portion of the weight lost, and a few may even regain it all.

Surgery usually improves most obesity-related complications such as type 2 diabetes mellitus, high blood pressure, heart failure, sleep apnea, etc. Blood sugar levels in many diabetics may even become normal, as may also happen with blood pressure in hypertensive patients and cholesterol/triglyceride levels in those who suffer from dyslipidemia.

It should be noted that there are significant risks in surgical intervention. Up to 10-20% of patients may require follow-up operations to correct complications of surgical intervention. Abdominal hernias as a result of wound separation following traditional open surgery are commonplace but less common in individuals when laparoscopic surgery is used. Breakdown of the gastric staple or suture lines with leakage, or stretched stomach pouch outlets reducing food restriction to less useful degrees, also may occur.

More than one third of patients develop gallstones believed to be due to rapid and substantial weight loss produced. Gallstones may be prevented with supplemental bile salts taken for the first 6 months post surgery, or the gallbladder may be removed prophylactically at the time of the surgical procedure.

Up to 30% of patients develop nutritional deficiencies such as anemia and osteopenia/osteoporosis which usually can be prevented with supplements.

Women of childbearing age should avoid pregnancy after surgery until weight loss becomes maximal and stable because rapid weight loss and nutritional deficiencies may harm a developing fetus/unborn child.

Death is reported to occur in less than 0.5% of cases.

Well-controlled clinical trials are needed before one can determine which surgical procedure is most effective and safe, and may be best to employ in any given patient or set of circumstances. Until this evidence is available, the choice of surgical procedure remains empirical. However, REY-GP appears to be an effective procedure most commonly employed in university centers

It should be recognized that there are no guarantees regarding treatment of overweight/obesity, surgery included, to produce weight loss and maintain it safely and effectively. Changes in lifestyle, diet, exercise, and behavior modification in a life-long program also remain essential for success.

For additional information, consult:

National Institute of Diabetes and Digestive and Kidney Diseases
(NIDDK)
* Report on: *Gastric Surgery for Severe Obesity*
  http://www.niddk.nih.gov/health/nutrit/pubs/gastsurg.htm

American Society for Bariatric Surgery
* Report on: *Rationale for the Treatment of Morbid Obesity*
  http://www.asbs.org/html/rationale/rationale.html

Obesity Treatment Center—UMDNJ—The University Hospital
* Report on: *What About Gastric Banding?*
  http://www.theuniversityhospital.com/otc/html/thesurgicalop-
  tion/gastricband.htm
* Report on: *See a Surgery: Vertical Banded Gastroplasty: Roux-En-Y
  Gastric Bypass: A Step-by-Step Approach*
  http://www.theuniversityhospital.com/otc/html/seeasurgery

Johns Hopkins Bayview Medical Center
* Report on: *Gastric Bypass Surgery for Obesity: Roux-En-Y Gastric
  Bypass*
  http://www.jhbmc.jhu.edu (search "obesity surgery")

American College of Surgeons
* Report on: *Recommendations for Facilities Performing Bariatric Surgery*
  http://www.facs.org/fellows_info/statements/st-34.html

National Heart, Lung, and Blood Institute
* Report on: *Guidelines on Overweight and Obesity: Electronic
  Textbook: Surgery for Weight Loss*
  http://www.nhlbi.nih.gov/guidelines/obestiy/e_txtbk/txgd/4326.htm

8. Searching the Web

Many books have been written on how to use/search the Internet/Web and obtain health information. You can obtain a book of your choice from your local public library or bookstore. If you already have one, use it accordingly. Or you can use the one recently published by the author entitled: "Web Health Information Resource Guide: For Consumers, Healthcare Providers, Patients and Physicians" published in 2001 by Author's Choice Press, iuniverse.com. The Web page for the book is: http://www.webspaner.com/users/webhealthdoc.

A number of commercial services such as AOL, MSN, Netscape, Yahoo, and Road Runner, as well as others, provide easy, reliable, and relatively inexpensive access to the Internet/Web via your computer. If you do not have a computer, you can use one at your local public, college or university library, and connect to the Internet/Web at no cost to you and little effort on your part. And, your local reference librarian can show you how to use/search the Web properly to facilitate your search. Should a computer not be available to you, or if you prefer, a Web TV or similar device hooked up to your TV set at home can connect you to the Internet/Web. Once connected, you are ready to start searching using the Author's List of Key Web Resources provided in Chapter 9. These Web resources are arranged alphabetically for ease of reference and each provides an outline of types of reports/information available.

Not all information made available on the Web should be considered current, comprehensive, reliable and useful. Therefore, you are cautioned to be selective and use due diligence in your search and use of information obtained. A good way to select appropriate Web resources is to use reliable guidelines in choosing them. Such guidelines may be obtained from a number of sources such as:

American Medical Association
http://www.ama-assn.org/ama/pub/category/1905.html

Health on the Net Foundation
http://www.hon.ch (click on "HON Code of Conduct")

Criteria used by different organizations in selecting Web resources varies. Nevertheless, using the guidelines developed by the above mentioned organizations and others should enable you to find Web resource information needed for your purpose.

The Author's List of Key Web Resources in Chapter 9 is a personally reviewed selection. They are regarded generally as providing the information needed on overweight, obesity and health-related complications for the vast majority of consumers, healthcare providers, patients and physicians.

The World Wide Web currently is estimated at well over 2 billion pages and 3 billion documents, and is still growing rapidly each day. When you search the Web with a search engine such as Google or AlltheWeb, etc., you are not searching it directly as this is not possible at this time. The Web is the totality of all the Web pages and documents that reside on computers, call servers, worldwide, and your computer cannot locate and search them directly. All you can do with your computer is to go to one of a number of intermediate resources that contain selected and organized Web pages and databases. Thus, via Google, for example, you merely search these intermediate resources/databases and they provide you with the links to the web pages needed to complete your search. You can then click on their links/Web pages and retrieve reports/documents/information pertaining to your particular search.

Google or AlltheWeb can provide you with a reasonably complete search on topics of interest, usually in less than a second or so. However, then you are left with the very difficult task of reviewing all the links/Web pages/reports/information found in order to find the ones that are current, comprehensive, reliable, and useful and meet your needs. This is not only difficult and time consuming but also usually well beyond the capability of most readers to do alone in a reasonable period of time.

To simplify matters for you, the author has personally and carefully selected and assembled the Author's List of Key Web Resources and listed them alphabetically for ease of reference, along with their Web sites, in Chapter 9.

For a general or a specific topic search regarding overweight, obesity and health-related complications, four reasonably good places to start your search are:

Medlineplus
http://www.nlm.nih.gov/medlineplus

National Institutes of Health
http://www.health.nih.gov

Intellihealth
http://www.intellihealth.com

WebMD
http://www.webmd.com

The above four are the Author's choice of Web Resources that serve as a starting point or general searches regarding overweight, obesity, and health-related complications information.

The main content of each of the Web Resources in the Author's List has been organized into categories, topics, and reports to facilitate your selection of those most likely to provide you with the information you may need. And, the Search site provided by each of these Web Resources may be used to obtain additional information on topics of interest from their database.

In the event you cannot easily find the appropriate Web Resource that may contain the information you are looking for, you can use the Search site on one or more of the U.S. Government or other web resources to search for and obtain available information.

Remember that the web is growing rapidly. As a result, it is in a constant state of flux, updating, and reorganization. Web Resources may change their names and/or Web addresses, formats, content and categorization of information offered. If for any reason the Web site you choose from the Author's List doesn't work for you when you try to connect, search the Web Resource name itself. If you still have problems connecting, try another Search Engine or an alternative Web Resource from the Author's List.

Keep in mind that various Web Resources use different methods to search the Web to compile their databases and information offered. Also, each organizes and categorizes information differently, some better than others. Thus, searches using different Web Resources or topics may provide results that differ and need to be reconciled.

For the most part, the information you find via the Author's List likely will be reasonably current, comprehensive, reliable and useful in most respects, but not necessarily all. Thus, you should not necessarily believe all information you obtain from any one Web Resource. Unlike medical/scientific articles published in peer reviewed professional journals, there is no guarantee that the information you obtain from any Web Resource will meet your needs in all respects. Also, keep in mind that Web Resources are not uniformly reliable in all aspects of all information offered. Therefore, it is suggested that you select and chose Web Resources that you feel are most appropriate for your purpose and compare and contrast information obtained from at least 2-3 or more different ones before reaching any conclusions/decisions in consultation with your physician/healthcare provider. Even in the world of the Web, a second and even a third opinion, is considered to be worthwhile.

One also needs to consider that even in the case of evidence-based information from well-controlled clinical trials, there are problems in terms of what the data collected and the study results mean. Clinical study evidence necessarily is subject to interpretation and application and as such is a subjective process. All of us are biased to some degree in one way or another not only in obtaining, but also in interpreting and applying information, evidence-based or not. Words, phrases, statistics, conclusions, etc. mean different things to different people at different times and places, depending on "where one is coming from". For example, even in the case of a long-standing document such as the Constitution of the United States, written by "great minds", lawyers, judges, and even the Supreme Court continue to argue about, and have great difficulty interpreting and applying, the so-called "original intent" of our founding fathers who authored the document.

Finally, you should note that not all information about overweight, obesity and health-related complications, advocated at any time will necessarily prove to be as reliable and useful as claimed. The history of overweight, obesity and health-related complications is replete with examples of past information and treatments, etc., advocated by leading figures of the time, that have turned out not to be very reliable or useful at all. Thus, "buyer beware".

Nevertheless, available evidence indicates that there are significant improvements in our understanding of causes, prevention, diagnosis, and treatment of overweight, obesity and health-related complications. The point now has been reached where overweight, obesity and health-related complications may be successfully treated in many cases. Understanding and treatment methods used are constantly improving and new advances are being made daily. Therefore, take charge, control and responsibility for your health and become informed.

9.   Author's List of Key Web Resources

9.1   AlltheWeb (FastSearch)
http://www.alltheweb.com

AlltheWeb is powered by Fast Search and Transfer (FAST) and now reports having over 2 billion documents in their Web catalog. It is regarded by many as one of the largest and best world-wide search engines.

FAST, founded in 1997, is headquartered in Oslo, Norway and has operations in the United States, Europe (Norway, Germany, Italy and the United Kingdom), and Japan. Visit http://www.fastsearch.com for additional information.

Examples of links and information featured after searching of the topic "obesity" include:

- ACERO Home page—latest news on obesity research
- American Obesity Association—comprehensive obesity information
- American Society of Bariatric Physicians—treatment of obesity (bariatrics)
- Association for the Study of Obesity
- Association for Morbid Obesity Support
- Childhood and Adolescent obesity
- Health and Obesity
- International Obesity Task Force
- Michael D. Meyers, M.D.—comprehensive overweight/obesity information
- Minnesota Obesity Center—nutrition research center
- Multi-Disciplinary Forum for Research and Treatment of Obesity
- NAASO: North American Association for the Study of Obesity
- NIDDK Health Information—weight loss and control information
- Obesity and Health—as little as a 10% weight loss improves an obese patient's health and lowers the risk of diabetes and heart disease
- Obesity and Diabetes –obesity and juvenile diabetes
- Obesity Law and Advocacy Center
- Obesity Treatment Center—UMDNJ University Hospital—for severely obese
- Obesity Virus—are some forms of obesity caused by a virus infection?
- Surgical Centers—for the treatment of severe obesity
- Stomach Banding—for severe obesity
- Weight Loss Programs and Management.

Search results are provided in a number of languages. Use the Search site to obtain additional information.

9.2 American Academy of Family Physicians (AAFP) http://www.aafp.org

The AAFP is one of the largest professional medical organizations, representing more than 90,000 family physicians nationwide. Founded in 1947, AAFP's mission is to preserve and promote the science and art of family medicine, and to ensure high-quality, cost-effective health care for patients. Family Practice is the medical specialty that provides comprehensive health care integrating biological, clinical and behavioral sciences.

Searching the topic of "obesity", links to the following reports are available:

• *Obesity: Assessment and Management in Primary Care*

Basic treatment of overweight and obese patients requires a comprehensive approach involving diet and nutrition, regular physical activity and behavioral change with emphasis on long-term weight management. Physicians and other health professionals play an important role in encouraging positive lifestyle behaviors as well as treating obesity-related diseases and counseling patients about safe and effective weight loss and weight maintenance programs.

This report provides information on:
• definition of overweight and obesity
• recommended average daily energy allowances for children and adults, body mass index calculation, measures of fatness, and waist circumference criteria
• epidemiology
• calculating daily caloric requirements
• disease risk associated with overweight and obesity by body mass index criteria
• expert guidance for the evaluation and management

- physical and psychological complications
- factors to consider when evaluating disease risk status in adults
- flow chart for treatment
- physician's role
- recommendations for adult weight loss therapy
- over all recommendations

- *Medical Management of Obesity*

Classifications of overweight and obesity in adults is given as:

Class	BMI
Normal	up to 24.9
Overweight	25.0-29.9
Obese	30.0 or greater

Patients in overweight and obesity classes usually may accomplish desired weight loss with diet, exercise, behavior and lifestyle modifications, particularly if they are not severely obese (BMI >40). Weight loss medications may be considered appropriate as adjuncts in selected patients, chiefly for short-term use. However, drugs are not designed to replace diet, exercise, and lifestyle modifications. Information is provided on:

- definitions of overweight and obesity
- body mass index chart
- classification of overweight and obesity in adults
- risk factors associated with increased morbidity and mortality
- etiology
- flow chart for management
- medications: basics, pros and cons
- new weight loss medications
- surgical interventions
- key references

• *Drug Therapy for Obesity*

Numerous strategies are available for the treatment of obesity. Behavioral therapy, adoption of healthy lifestyle, regular exercise, diet, counseling, medical management, surgical, and drug (pharmacologic) treatment all have been used with varying degrees of success, and continues to offer the basis for the best treatment for long-term weight loss and maintenance. Anorectic drugs offer only limited additional benefit for most patients

A chart of drugs approved by the FDA for the treatment of obesity is provided giving the name of the agent, proposed mechanism of action, dosage, potential drug interactions and possible adverse effects, etc. The report further advises that all of the drugs presently available appear to produce similar moderate degrees of weight loss and the choice of drug for any given patient is largely empiric in most cases.

Use Search site for additional information.

9.3   American Academy of Pediatrics (AAP)
http://www.aap.org

The AAP was founded at Harper Hospital in Detroit in 1930. Since then, the AAP has grown to a membership of more than 53,000 primary care pediatricians, pediatric medical sub-specialists, and pediatric surgical specialists. The mission of the AAP is to attain optimal physical, mental, and social health and well-being for all infants, children, adolescents and young adults.

Searching the topic "obesity", links/information are available on:
• study focusing on predictors of adult obesity
• obesity related to youths aged 6-17
• rise in childhood obesity and type 2 diabetes

- management of child and adolescent obesity
- racial divergence in adiposity during adolescence
- effects of metformin on body mass index and glucose tolerance in obese adolescents
- list of nutrition information
- federal health officials support use of newer growth charts
- food safety for children
- adult food fears impact children
- healthy lifestyles study to assess the effectiveness of an office-based intervention to improve eating and activity patterns and stabilize weight gain of children at risk for obesity
- care for the adolescent—addresses key medical and parental concerns about nutrition
- TV encourages poor lifestyle choices

Use the Search site to obtain additional information.

9.4　American Association of Clinical Endocrinologists (AACE)—American College of Endocrinology (ACE) http://www.aace.com/college

AACE/ACE was founded in 1991 and has over 4,000 members throughout the United States and in 63 foreign countries dedicated to the principles of patient care, education, and clinical research. Its mission is to provide and promote education, research, and communication in the art and science of clinical endocrinology, and promote appropriate recognition of advances and achievements relating to the field.

Searching the topic "obesity", a report entitled *AACE/ACE Position Statement Regarding the Prevention, Diagnosis, and Treatment of Obesity* (1998 Revision) is made available. This report provides information on:

- introduction
- definition
- etiology and pathogenesis
  - physiologic-genetic mechanism
  - genetic predisposition
  - low energy output
  - regulation of peptides and neurotransmitters
  - hypothalamic abnormalities
  - environmental mechanisms
  - drugs
  - social factors
  - high energy and fat intake
  - inactivity
  - psychological factors
- associated health risks
  - diabetes mellitus, type 2
  - cardiovascular disease
  - essential hypertension
  - stroke
  - cardiomyopathy
  - coronary heart disease
  - atherosclerosis
  - reproductive disorders
  - endometrial cancer
  - breast cancer
  - colon cancer
  - prostate cancer
  - gallbladder disease
  - respiratory disease
  - psychological disorders
  - weight cycling
  - other co-morbidities

- prevention
- risk factors
- diagnosis
- weight management strategies
  - basic treatment
  - lifestyle changes/behavior modification
  - physical activity
  - pharmacotherapy
  - weight loss
  - maintenance of weight loss
  - recommended use of available agents
  - other products
  - surgical treatment
- pediatric and adolescent obesity
  - associated health risk
  - risk factors
  - diagnosis
  - weight management strategies

Use the Search site to obtain additional information.

9.5   American College of Cardiology (ACC)
http://www.acc.org

ACC has a membership of around 26,000 including cardiologists from the U.S. and around the world. Members are dedicated to providing optimal cardiovascular care and easy access to timely, sought-after information. ACC's *Guidelines Applied in Practice Programs* is an effort to improve the quality of cardiovascular care by bringing ACC/AHA (American Heart Association) practice guidelines to the point of care.

Searching the topic "obesity", links/information available include:
- assessment of cardiovascular risk
- perioperative cardiovascular evaluation update
- exercise testing guidelines
- coronary artery bypass graft surgery guidelines
- junk food
- news releases

Use the Search site to obtain additional information.

9.6 American College of Physicians— American Society of Internal Medicine (ACP-ASIM) http://www.acponline.org

The ACP-ASIM is the nation's largest medical specialty society with approximately 115,000 members. Its mission is to enhance the effectiveness of health care by fostering excellence and professionalism in the practice of internal medicine.

Searching "obesity" links/information include:
- role of drugs in treating obesity
- physical activity, obesity, and the risk for colon cancer and adenoma
- obesity as an adverse prognostic factor for patients receiving adjuvant chemotherapy for breast cancer
- most obesity treatment methods are ineffective over the long term
- sleep disorders and obesity hypoventilation: when to suspect and how to manage
- prescription weight loss pills in the treatment of obese persons with a body mass index of 30 or higher or 27 plus an obesity-related complications
- men with type 2 diabetes or impaired glucose tolerance and risk of early death

- serum insulin levels associated with hypertension
- orlistat and diet, effective and safe for weight loss and coronary risk reduction
- relation between plasma leptin levels, body fat, and obesity
- natural history of the development of obesity in young adults
- obesity and end-of-life care
- role of leptin in human obesity
- understanding the complex journey to obesity
- obesity and complications after diet or exercise-induced weight loss in men
- prevalence of obesity, contribution of physical activity and genetic factors
- obesity and reasons to change behavior
- screening for cervical and breast cancer –obesity as an unrecognized barrier
- obesity is important in understanding occurrence of cancer
- type 2 diabetes is associated with low birth weight followed by obesity
- insulin resistance and obesity
- obesity and hypertension
- sleep apnea is 10 to 20 times more common in men
- BMI 30 or more is associated with a particularly high risk for type 2 diabetes
- snoring behavior, wake time sleepiness and fatigue indicates high risk for sleep apnea
- obesity and rapid weight loss are risk factors for cholesterol gallstones
- National Task Force for the Prevention and Treatment of Obesity and Weight Cycling
- diet and weight loss are important steps in the management of type 2 diabetes

- continuous and intermittent sibutramine appears to be equally effective
- glucose levels are associated with cardiovascular risk
- regular exercise is associated with a reduced incidence of diabetes mellitus
- physical activity is associated with lower risk of breast cancer
- high waist-to-hip ratio increases risk of death
- anorectic medications enhanced weight-loss programs
- dietary strategies alone reduce weight in non insulin-dependent diabetes
- weight loss in obese patients with asthma improves lung function
- obesity, hypertension, and the risk of kidney cancer

Use Search site for additional information.

9.7 American College of Rheumatology (ACR) http://www.rheumatology.org

The ACR is the professional organization dedicated to healing of, and preventing disability from, various forms of arthritis involving the joints, muscles, and bone.

Osteoarthritis and gouty arthritis, are recognized complications of overweight and obesity.

Searching the topic "obesity and arthritis", reports available include:
- *Recommendations for the Medical Management of Osteoarthritis of the Hip and Knee*
  http://www.rheumatology.org/research/guidelines/oa-mgmt/oa-mgmt.html
- *Exercise and Arthritis*
  http://www.rheumatology.org/patients/factsheet/exercise.html

- *Gouty Arthritis*
  http://www.rheumatology.org/publications/primarycare/
  number4/hrh0021498.html

Physically active people generally are healthier and live longer than those who remain sedentary and largely inactive. Certain kinds of physical activity may produce important benefits in patients with arthritis. Furthermore, it should be recognized that patients with arthritis can safely participate in appropriate regular exercise programs and achieve better aerobic, muscular and cardiovascular fitness. Low impact exercises, such as swimming and water aerobics may be particularly well-tolerated by people with arthritis. Improved strength, endurance, and flexibility and better ability to walk or perform daily tasks are all benefits of exercise/physical activity.

Three main types of exercise may play a role in maintaining or improving health and fitness, in patients with osteoarthritis and gout, and reducing arthritis-related pain and discomfort and disability. These include:

- flexibility or stretching—low intensity daily exercises to maintain or improve range of motion of joints in the arms, legs, neck and back are the basis of most therapeutic exercise programs. Greater flexibility generally improves function, decreases pain and discomfort, improves motion/tasks, and reduces the chance for injuries.
- muscle conditioning—strength and endurance exercises which are more vigorous than flexibility/stretching exercises. These are usually done every other day to give the body a chance to recuperate between sessions. Lifting the weight of the arms, legs or trunk against gravity, or using weights, elastic bands or weight/muscle building machines for more resistance, all enable muscles, ligaments and joints work harder and longer.

- aerobic cardio-respiratory conditioning exercises improve heart, lung and muscle function as well as range of motion and joint mobility decreasing progression of arthritis as well as pain and discomfort.

A comprehensive exercise program for a patient with arthritis may include flexibility as well as aerobic and strengthening activities. Content and progression of the patient's exercise program depends in a large measure on individual needs, capabilities, and the extent and degree of arthritis present. Those patients with long-standing or severe disease or multiple joint/site involvement should only consider undertaking an exercise program under the supervision of their physician/health care provider.

Use the Search site to obtain additional information.

9.8   American College of Surgeons (ACS) http://www.facs.org

ACS consists of specialists in surgery. It was founded in 1913 setting high standards for surgical education and practice. The letters FACS (Fellow American College of Surgeons) after a surgeon's name mean that education, training, professional qualifications, surgical competence and ethical conduct have passes a rigorous evaluation and have been found to be consistent with the standards established.

A key ACS report is provided on surgical treatment of severe obesity is entitled: (ST-34) *Recommendations for Facilities Performing Bariatric Surgery* available at:
http://www.facs.org/fellows_info/statements/st-34.html

Severe (massive) or morbid obesity is defined by ACS as more than 100 pounds greater than normal body weight or a body mass index (BMI) greater than 40 (>35 if associated with significant complications). Five percent or more of the US population, or around 15 million persons, are estimated to suffer from severe obesity at this time.

ACS states that diet or drug therapy programs are reported to consistently yield disappointing results, and have failed to bring about significant, sustained weight loss in the majority of severely obese patients. However, ACS believe that morbid obesity can be effectively treated with established surgical procedures, achieving substantial weight reduction and improved quality of life in the majority of patients with "acceptable" rates of mortality and morbidity. Optimal environment for achieving good outcome is stated to be a well-prepared and committed surgeon, an established and experienced bariatric surgical team, appropriate institutional/hospital resources and equipment, and a comprehensive system for satisfactory patient evaluation and follow-up.

Well-controlled trials remain to be conducted to compare various surgical procedures and to establish the efficacy, safety and role of surgery versus medical treatment of severe obesity.

Use the Search site to obtain additional information.

9.9 American Diabetes Association (ADA)
http://www.diabetes.org

ADA provides diabetes research information and advocacy. Its mission is to improve the lives of all people affected, and eventually to help find a "cure" for diabetes mellitus. To fulfill this mission, the ADA funds research, publishes scientific findings, and provides information and other services to patients, their families, health care professionals and the public. ADA also is actively involved in advocating for scientific research and for the rights of patients with diabetes.

In 1998, the National Institutes of Health published evidence-based *Clinical Guidelines on the Identification, Evaluation and Treatment of Overweight and Obesity in Adults* using body mass index (BMI) criteria. As such, a BMI lower than 18.5 constitutes underweight; 18.5-24.9=normal weight; 25-29.9=overweight; 30-34.9=mild obesity; 35-39.9=moderate obesity; and 40.0 or higher=severe obesity. Overweight and obese categories represent increasing disease risk for complications such as type 2 diabetes mellitus, hypertension, and cardiovascular disease relative to normal weight. Waist circumference is directly correlated with abdominal fat and higher risk for type 2 diabetes mellitus and cardiovascular disease, etc. .

Two key links and reports are made available using the Search site and the topic "obesity":
* *Obesity Overview*
* *The Role of Exercise in the Treatment of Obesity*

The *Obesity Overview* report points out that:
* overweight and obesity represent a major public health concern
* approximately 54% of adults aged 20 years or older are affected
* there is increased risk of morbidity from type 2 diabetes, hypertension, dyslipidemia, coronary heart disease, stroke, gout, sleep apnea, gallbladder disease, osteoarthritis, and some forms of cancer
* increase in obesity has occurred in both sexes and all major racial/ethnic groups
* weight loss in overweight or obese individuals decreases risk factors for diabetes mellitus and cardiovascular disease
* provides NIH published *Clinical Guidelines on the Identification, Evaluation and Treatment of Overweight and Obesity in Adults*

- a public health problem exists in US children—1 in 5 are overweight (or obese)
- BMI may not be appropriate for children and adolescents
- overweight during childhood/adolescence is associated with overweight in adulthood
- treatment of obesity for long lasting change is difficult at best
- clearly developed healthy lifestyle patterns in patients is essential
- prevention and treatment require a multi-disciplined, multi-targeted approach

The Role of Exercise in the Treatment of Obesity report points out that:
- exercise, diet and behavioral modification/education are typically prescribed concurrently as first order treatment of overweight and obesity
- aerobic and resistance exercise are the two modalities found to be useful for treating individuals who are overweight
- aerobic exercise training is used to help establish a negative energy balance and drive the metabolic processes that may help to decrease body weight
- aerobic exercise is known to promote the use of fat as a fuel and promote fat oxidation in obese men and women when combined with a low fat calorie reduced diet
- aerobic exercise combined with a balanced calorie-reduced diet also has been shown to increase fat oxidation in obese men and women at risk for type 2 diabetes mellitus
- exercise/diet programs also lead to an improvement in insulin sensitivity which is related to changes in body composition, specifically a loss of visceral fat
- resistance exercise can increase muscle mass and has been shown to increase resting metabolism

- studies in obese women have shown that resistance exercise coupled with dietary restriction produces a greater decrease in resting metabolism compared to aerobic exercise.

Use the Search site to obtain additional information.

9.10   American Heart Association (AHA)
http://www.americanheart.org

AHA is a large lay and professional organization devoted to cardiovascular disease. Their national center is located in Dallas, Texas, with 15 affiliate offices scattered throughout the USA. Combined efforts involve the work of millions of volunteers and supporters dedicated to the primary task of reducing disability and death from cardiovascular disease and strokes.

Searching the topic, "obesity", the following key links/information, are made available:
- obesity and overweight
- AHA guidelines for weight management programs for healthy adults
- dietary guidelines for healthy american adults
- understanding obesity in youth
- kids getting a steady diet of fast food on the TV
- your kids are what you eat
- dietary guidelines for healthy children
- response to high-fat, low-carbohydrate weight loss diets
- dietary guidelines
- diet and nutrition
- dietary recommendations
- alcohol, wine and cardiovascular disease
- step I and step II diets

- fad diets
- fiber, lipids and coronary heart disease
- dietary/weight loss supplements
- anti-obesity drug link to valve disease confirmed
- slowing excess weight gain in childhood appears to reduce adult heart disease risk
- obesity impact on cardiovascular disease
- Mexican Americans more likely to die of heart disease
- be smart for your heart
- diabetes is a major risk factor for heart disease and stroke
- women and cardiovascular disease
- women and children face the music of the deadly quartet
- Syndrome X
- lifestyle and diet changes prevent coronary heart disease, obesity hurts
- risk factors I can change
- healthy life style
- physical inactivity, overweight and obesity
- exercise (physical activity) is beneficial for older people with disabilities
- exercise (physical activity) and children
- physical activity may reduce levels of "fat hormone" in men
- patients and physical activity
- body composition and why it is important
- high blood pressure gene linked to obesity

Use the Search site to obtain additional information.

9.11 American Hiking Society (AHS)
http://www.americanhiking.org

AHS is dedicated to serving hikers and protecting the nation's hiking trails and surrounding environment. A healthy hiking vacation and/or joining a trail club to get outside and hike, and enjoy the scenic outdoors with other like-minded individuals is an excellent way to engage in useful physical activity/exercise, and get involved in conservation and support of protecting our nation's scenic and historic trails and surrounding environment.

Find out about:
- alliance of hiking organizations
- events and volunteer opportunities
- hiker's emporium
- hiker's info center
- inside American hiking
- join American hiking
- news and resources
- trail conservation and policy

9.12 American Medical Association (AMA)
http://www.ama-assn.org

The AMA is one of the nation's leaders in promoting professionalism in medicine and setting standards for medical practice and ethics. Its mission is to promote the science and art of medicine and the betterment of public health. The Consumer Health Information site allows one to learn how to improve their health with easy-to-understand, high-quality health information for the patient.

Obtain the latest on research and other developments on overweight, obesity and health from JAMA (the Journal of the AMA), Archives of Internal Medicine, Archives of General Psychiatry and American Medical News, publications of AMA.

Searching the topic "obesity", links/information include:
- overweight, obesity and health risk
- diet and exercise in the treatment of obesity
- role of the prenatal environmental in the development of obesity
- a weight matter: obesity, leptin, and beyond
- treating the obese patient
- weighing options: the business of helping obese patients
- dieting and the development of eating disorders
- leptin and reproduction
- adiposity and coronary heart disease in women
- lifestyle activity versus structured aerobic exercise in obese women
- diabetes mellitus and cardiovascular disease in women
- effects of intermittent exercise and use of home exercise equipment
- walking, vigorous physical activity, and type 2 diabetes in women
- screening for cervical and breast cancer in obesity
- effect of maternal obesity on perinatal morbidity
- effects of smoking and obesity on asthma among women
- relationship between obesity and breast cancer
- adult options for childhood obesity
- cutting the fat: CDC report targets childhood obesity
- treating the obese patient

Use the Search site to obtain additional information.

9.13 American Obesity Association (AOA)
   http://www.obesity.org

AOA's Board of Directors, and Advisory Council are composed of leading researchers and clinicians in the field of obesity. AOA regards obesity as not a simple case of eating too much but rather as a serious chronic disease. It states that no condition—not race, religion, gender, or other disease compares to obesity in prevalence and prejudice, mortality and morbidity, sickness and stigma.

AOA provides links/information on:
*   education
*   research
*   prevention
*   treatment
*   consumer protection
*   discrimination
*   childhood obesity
*   disability due to obesity
*   professional member directory
*   fast facts
*   editorial
*   news

Use the Search site for additional information.

9.14 American Society for Bariatric Surgery (ASBS)
   http://www.asbs.org

Founded in 1983, ASBS specializes in bariatric (obesity) surgery. It is a founding member of the International Federation for the Surgery of Obesity (IFSO). ASBS members automatically become members of IFSO.

Bariatric Surgery is a recognized sub-specialty in the field of General Surgery. It is a specialty surgical society in the Specialty and Service Society of the American Medical Association. Regular members of ASBS are all Board Certified Surgeons who have a special interest in the surgical treatment of severely obese patients.

Information sites featured include:
- organization of ASBS
- rational for surgery
- story of surgery for obesity
- find members in your area
- calculate your body mass index
- related sites of interest
- Journal Obesity Surgery
- guidelines

A report entitled: *Rational for the Surgical Treatment of Morbid Obesity*, (2001) is made available and provides a detailed summary report on:
- introduction
- rationale for the surgical treatment of severe obesity
- non-operative treatment
- surgical treatment guide
- patient selection
- risk of surgical treatment
- International Bariatric Surgery Registry (IBSR)
  - results from IBSR pooled report
  - 30-day complication information
- results
- childbearing
- nutritional consequence of gastric restriction surgery for obesity
- specific recommendations can be made for the treatment of severe obesity

- preoperative psychological testing
- conclusions
- key literature references

The Introduction of the laproscopic approach to bariatric surgery is reported to offer improvement in patient comfort, length of hospital stay, and results. A report entitled: SAGES/ASBS *Guidelines for Laparoscopic and Conventional Surgical Treatment of Morbid Obesity* report is available at: http://asbs.org/html/guidelines.html

This reports provides information on:
- introduction
- indications for surgery
- peri-operative and long term management considerations
- surgical techniques
- summary
- key literature references

For additional information, consult:
http://www.obesityhelp.com/morbidobesity.

This site provides links/information on:
- pictures/explanations of bariatric surgical procedures used
- benefits and risks
- what to expect
- frequently asked questions/answers

9.15 CDC National Center for Chronic Disease Prevention and Health Promotion (NCCDPHP)
http://www.cdc.gov/nccdphp/dnpa
http://www.cdc.gov

CDC serves as the national focus for developing and applying disease prevention and control, environmental health, and health promotion and education activities designed to improve the health of people in the United States and abroad

One of the major CDC centers is the National Center for Chronic Disease Prevention and Health Promotion (NCCDPHP) which is dedicated to preventing premature death and disability from chronic diseases and promoting healthy personal behaviors. Overweight, obesity and health are prime interests and concern for the NCCDPHP.

The Division of Nutrition and Physical Activity (DNPA) at the CDC addresses the role of nutrition and physical activity in health promotion and the prevention and control of chronic disorders such as overweight and obesity. DNPA programs include epidemiology, applied research, public health policy, surveillance, community interventions, evaluation, and communications. It is organized into the: 1) Chronic Disease Nutrition Branch, 2) Maternal Nutrition Branch, and 3) Physical Activity and Health Branch, and 4) Related Information.

Key reports regarding overweight and obesity include:
*   *Obesity and Overweight: An Overview* http://www.cdc.gov/ nccdphp/dnpa/obesity/index.htm
*   *Body Mass Index (BMI)* http://www.cdc.gov/nccdphp/dnpa/obesity/bmi.htm
*   *Diet, Nutrition and Physical Activity* http://www.cdc.gov/nccdphp/dnpa
*   *Physical Activity: Ready Set* http://www.cdc.gov/nccdphp/dnpa/readyset/index.htm
*   *Physical Activity Evaluation Handbook* http://www.cdc.gov/ nccdphp/dnpa/physical/handbook/index.htm
*   *Physical Activity Recommendations* http://www.cdc.gov/nccdphp/dnpa/physical/recommendations.htm

- *Physical Activity Tips*
  http://www.cdc.gov/nccdphp/dnpa/phys_act.htm
- *Physical Activity Topics*
  http://www.cdc.gov/nccdphp/dnpa/physicalactivity.htm
- *PEP: A Personal Energy Plan*
  http://www.cdc.gov/nccdphp/dnpa/pep.htm
- *Healthy Eating Tips*
  http://www.cdc.gov/nccdphp/dnpa/heal_eat.htm
- *Five a Day: Fruits and Vegetables*
  http://www.cdc.gov/nccdphp/dnpa/5Aday.htm
- *ACEs: Active Community Environments*
  http://www.cdc.gov/nccdphp/dnpa/aces.htm
- *Kids Walk-to-School*
  http://www.cdc.gov/nccdphp/dnpa/kidswalk/index.htm

Use the Search site to obtain additional reports/information.

9.16   Cyberdiet (CD)
http://www.cyberdiet.com

Cyberdiet founded in 1995, joined the DietWatch.com network of diet and nutrition resources on the Internet. It is reported to average over 15 million visits a month, and to have received rave reviews from both visitors and the media.

Interactive Tools allow users to customize a diet and nutrition program to achieve their specific goals as well as to provide this information at the click of a mouse.

Featured sites include information on:
- getting started
- free personal profile

- eating right
- exercising smart
- feeling good
- community
- "nutritional profile" which produces nutrient requirements
- "assessment tools" with information about fat distribution
- "12-week meal plans" provides daily meals and calorie ranges, adjusted for particular lifestyle and personal considerations ranging from vegetarian to convenience food, along with shopping lists and recipes
- latest nutritional, exercise, and motivational information
- "food facts" provides answers to many questions about diet and nutrition
- "exercise tips" keeps users informed
- "help desk" provides added motivational advice needed to succeed
- "message forums" and "live chat room" for information and support
- "success stories" of dieters through healthy choices

9.17   Drug Info Net (DIN)
http://www.druginfonet.com

Drug Info Net provides information and links on "anti-obesity", "anorectic", and other drugs used in the treatment of overweight, obesity, and health-related complications. Featured sites include:

- drugs
- diseases
- pharmaceutical manufacturer's information
- healthcare news
- health
- healthcare.org
- government sites
- medical reference

- hospitals on-line
- medical schools on-line

Information is made available on overweight and obesity, eating disorders, medical complications, by Michael D. Meyers, M.D., concerning:
- definition
- prevalence
- diagnostic criteria
- eating behaviors and mood
- patient education
- psychological factors
- medical complications
- treatments
- weight loss gimmicks
- frequently asked questions
- health and sciences TV obesity program

Prevalence of obesity in the United States is based on the Behavior Risk Factor Surveillance System (BRFSS), a random digit dialed telephone survey of adults in the United States, courtesy of the Center for Disease Control and Prevention (CDC).

Drug information provided includes FDA Official Package Inserts for anti-obesity/anorectic drugs, as well as Patient Package Inserts for both health professionals and consumers. These are made available by brand name, generic name, manufacturer, and therapeutic class for all anorectic and other drugs used in the treatment of overweight and obesity.

Use the Search site to obtain additional reports/information.

9.18   Duke Diet and Fitness Center (DDFC)
http://www.dukecenter.org

The Duke University Health System is regarded as one of America's oldest and most successful weight management centers. Their program includes healthy eating, regular physical activity, stress management, and adherence to practical medical advice. DDFC does not offer any magic cure for overweight or obesity but rather an opportunity to take control of your life with positive long-term beneficial changes in many cases. The program is for adults 18 years of age and older.

Basic program includes:
*   nutrition: smart choices
    Meals are low in calories, fat, and sodium. Weekly nutrition lectures and group workshops teach a healthy, low fat, meal plan and how to make smart choices when dining out. Survival skills taught include restaurant field trips and grocery store shopping tours.
*   fitness: exercise
    Regular exercise is considered essential for weight control and a healthy lifestyle. Instruction is provided on how to exercise effectively and safely. The exercise plan is designed to produce desired weight loss, help strengthen muscles and improve balance, coordination, and flexibility. Physical activity includes water aerobics, strength and flexibility, and lap swimming for endurance. Gym activities include aerobics, yoga, tai chi, stretching and strength training using a broad range of fitness equipment, weight machines, free weights, treadmills, bicycles, rowing machines, and stair-climbing machines. Outdoor walking is encouraged in good weather on the nearby Duke University campus.
*   health psychology: reach your goals
    Clinical psychologists and social workers teach practical techniques and strategies for stress reduction, lifelong weight management,

changes in unhealthy behaviors, motivation, building confidence for success, and how to reach goals.

- medical management
Comprehensive medical assessment and a management treatment program that meets patient needs and addresses not only diet, exercise, and weight loss but also the complications of obesity such as diabetes, hypertension, high cholesterol, heart disease, etc.
- support program
Companion, support, and lifestyle maintenance programs are provided for long term management and success.

Participation in the DDFC program may be regarded as on the expensive side. Thus, DDFC is probably not for the average obese person even though past participants appear to speak highly about the program and results obtained.

9.19   eFit (Nutricise.com) http://www.efit.com

eFit/Nutricise.com was created with the goal of helping people lose weight, get in shape, and achieve the body that they want and deserve. Commitment to these goals resulted in the Nutricise Weight Loss Program. This program combines nutrition, exercise, and behavior modification with a personalized one-on-one nutritional coach for effective and long lasting weight loss results

The Nutricise team is comprised of experts in the fields of nutrition, exercise, behavior modification and motivational psychology/science. Nutritionists are American Dietetic Association Registered Dieticians.

Key information sites featured include:
- channels
  - cardio fitness
  - cooking and nutrition
  - cycling
  - diet and weight loss
  - fit style
  - golf
  - healthy living
  - running
  - snow sports
  - strength training
  - swimming
  - tennis
  - walking and hiking
  - women's health
  - yoga and mind-body
- healthy living tools
  - activity calorie counter
  - body mass index
  - fitness calculator
  - food nutrition search
  - gym locator
  - healthy restaurant locator
- custom program
  - free personal meal plan
  - free personal exercise plan
- community
  - share weight loss tips
  - buddy board
  - exercise and fitness
  - food and mood

- healthy living portal
  - alternative medicine
  - fitness
  - food and thought
  - health
  - healthy living shopping
  - mind and body
  - sports and recreation

For additional information, consult:
http://www.nutricise.com/newsite/what_is,html

9.20 Endocrine Society (ES)
http://www.endo-society.org

Founded in 1916, ES is internationally known as a leading source of state-of-the art research and clinical advancements in endocrinology and metabolism. It is dedicated to promoting excellence in research, education, and clinical practice in the field of endocrinology, and includes an international body of more than 9,500 members from the fields of medicine, molecular and cellular biology, biochemistry, physiology, genetics, immunology, education, industry and allied health.

Searching the topic "obesity" links/information include:
- causes of obesity and possible treatments
- "functional foods" in the dietary management of obesity
- brain reception may play a role in obesity
- latest research in obesity
- obese children often become obese adults
- diabetes, obesity, Metabolic Syndrome X
- patients with cortisol excess develop central obesity

- estrogen receptor alpha regulates the effect of estrogen on metabolic rate and maybe involved in the development of obesity in post menopausal women and men
- leptin plays a role in appetite and weight regulation in humans
- ghrelin is involved in weight regulation

Use the Search site provided to obtain additional information.

9.21   First Gov (FG)
http://www.firstgov.gov

First Gov is the official gateway to all U.S. Government information on more than 51 million Web pages from federal and state governments, District of Columbia, and U.S. territories. It is an interagency initiative administered by the U.S. General Services Administration and went online September 2000. Most of its Web pages are not available via commercial channels. Therefore, First Gov provides the most comprehensive search of U.S. government health information anywhere on the Internet/Web.

For pertinent overweight, obesity and health information of interest, search the "Health and Safety" site. Health and Consumer Safety provides resources regarding health, diseases, drugs, food and consumer safety. Links/information sites featured include:
- general health
  - facts for you: health statistics and facts
  - fitness and sports
  - globalhealth.gov
  - health and disease information from the National Institutes of Health
  - health and medicine at science.gov
  - health data warehouse

- Healthfinder—health information guide
- Healthfinder en espanol
- Medlineplus—consumer health information
- U.S. Department of Health and Human Services
- by ethnic group
  - African American health
  - Asian American health
  - Hispanic American health
  - Native American health
- general food sites
  - consumer advice on food and nutrition
  - food advice from: consumer.gov
  - food at: science.gov
  - Food and Drug Administration
  - food publications
  - food safety
  - nutrition
- specific health topics
  - consumer health
  - diabetes
  - drugs and medicines via Medlineplus resources
  - disability
  - growth charts for children
  - health promotion and disease prevention
  - heart disease and cholesterol
  - mental health
  - neurological disorders and stroke
  - obesity
  - online check-ups
- health insurance
- state and local resources

"General Health", "General Food" and "Specific Health" sites provide useful links/information.

Use the Search site to obtain additional information.

9.22 Food and Drug Administration (FDA)
http://www.fda.gov

The FDA regulates food, nutrition, dietary supplements, prescription, over-the-counter and generic drugs, beginning with the 1906 Food and Drugs Act, 1938 Federal Food, Drug, and Cosmetics Act, and the 1962 Drug Amendments.

Food and nutrition are evaluated/regulated via the FDA Center for Food Safety and Applied Nutrition (CFSAN) (http://www.cfsan.fda.gov).

Prescription, over-the-counter, and generic drugs are regulated via the FDA Center for Drug Evaluation and Research. (http://www.fda.gov/cder)

Key links/information sites are provided for:
- safety alerts
- product approvals
- laws FDA enforces
- Federal Register

Searching "obesity drugs" and "anorectic drugs", links and information sites include:
- FDA announces withdrawal of fenfluramine and dexfenfluramine but not phentermine
- phen/fen and valvular heart disease
- orlistat (Xenical), a newer anti-obesity agent

- drugs should be used only in patients with significant obesity and not in those with minimal disease
- it has not been established that the action of anorectic drugs is primarily one of appetite suppression
- xenical, a lipase inhibitor, is now available to treat obesity
- organic causes of obesity (e.g., hypothyroidism, Cushing's Syndrome, etc.)
- use of thyroid hormone, alone or combined with other drugs is unjustified and ineffective in the treatment of obesity without hypothyroidism
- adult obese patients instructed in dietary management and treated with anorectic drugs lose more weight on average than on placebo

Use the Search site to obtain additional information.

9.23   FDA Center for Drug Evaluation and Research (CDER) http://www.fda.gov/cder

CDER is dedicated to improving public health and promoting safe and effective drug use. A "CDER Handbook" site describes the Center's processes and activities.

"FDA Consumer" site provides articles with information about CDER and prescription, over-the-counter and generic drugs as well as dietary supplements, etc. used in the treatment of overweight and obesity.

"FDA News" site covers latest information concerning press releases as well as additional information.

Other reports provided include: *From Test Tube to Patient: Improving Health through Human Drug and Managing the Risks of Medical Product Use: Creating a Risk Management Framework.*

Important CDER accomplishments can be found via the links/sites:
- CDER 2001 Report to the Nation: *Improving Public Health through Human Drugs*
- New Drug Approval Reports
- Office of Drug Safety Annual Report

Additional key links/information sites include:
- drug information
- regulatory guidance
- CDER calendar/archives
- new consumer information
- new over-the-counter medicine label
- generic drugs: questions and answers
- drug approvals
- stay informed: daily/weekly updates
- MedWatch—safety alerts for FDA regulated products

Searching the topic "anti-obesity drugs" reports include:
- *Xenical: First in a New Class of Non-Systemic Acting Anti-Obesity Drugs Known as Lipase Inhibitors*
- *Ways to Win at Weight Loss*
- *Warns Against Herbal Fen-Phen*
- *Prescription Anti-Obesity Drugs*
- *Approves Sibutramine to treat Obesity*
- *Losing Weight is More than Counting Calories*

Use Search site for additional information.

9.24   FDA Center for Food Safety and Applied Nutrition (CFSAN)
http://www.cfsan.fda.gov

The CFSAN Web site provides key information on food, nutrition, food labeling, food safety, and other important topics.

Key links/information sites featured include:
- what's new
- press announcements and fact sheets
- dietary supplements
- food labeling and nutrition
- selected topics: subject index
- other regulatory agencies with responsibilities for food
- www.foodsafety.gov (gateway to government food safety information)
- kids, teens, and educators
- selected health topics
- seniors
- women's health
- Code of Federal Regulations
- Federal Register documents
- laws enforced by FDA
- selected non-FDA sources of food and nutrition or chemical or biological information

Use the Search site for additional information.

9.25   Global Health and Fitness (GHF)
http://www.global-fitness.com

GHF provides health and fitness recommendations and tools, including personal consulting, customized programs, fitness tracking software, exercise instructions and video demonstrations—all in easy-to-understand, easy-to-follow formats. Ways are provided to help develop a program that is "right for you"—one that is realistic and effective for you, your fitness level and time commitment.

Click on "Site Map" for "Health and Fitness" links/information including:
- fitness analysis –receive a free, comprehensive, step-by-step plan on how to reach your goals
- five components of optimal health—GHF integrated program implements all 5 components in combinations that are "right" for you, namely:
  - strength training—exercise instructions, video demonstrations, and a detailed explanation of each muscle group, its location, and best exercises for the group
  - weight management—using GHF's *Weight Management Book*—a guide to adopting changes that make healthy eating and physical activity life-long pursuits—including recipes, healthy shopping list, and recipe search index
  - cardiovascular exercise—instruction and video demonstrations regarding 7 effective cardiovascular exercises
  - nutrition—guide, including food sources, easy-to-follow recommendations of 6 basic nutrients including the ratio of each for you to reach your fitness goal
  - flexibility training—flexibility exercises, instructions, and video demonstrations of 20 effective stretches, and a detailed explanation of each muscle group, its location, and the effective stretching exercise for that group
- *Secrets to Peak Performance*—book regarding fitness
- *Protrack*—fitness tracking software
- fitness tools including:
  - basal metabolic rate (BMR) calculator
  - body mass index (BMI) calculator

- calorie calculator
- protein calculator
- fat calculator
- carbohydrate calculator
- heart rate calculator
- nutritional food database
- waist-to-hip ratio calculator
- GHF membership includes:
  - fitness consulting—questions receive a response within 24 hours from experts
  - all programs customized for you
  - all 5 GHF online books free
  - hundreds of exercise instructions and video demonstrations
  - healthy recipes and meal plans
  - full retail version of Protrack—helps members keep detailed records of workouts, measurements (e.g., body fat, or waist size) and nutritional information while allowing one to print and analyze this information and reports with one's computer
  - motivational and latest fitness research information sent free
  - special discounts at one of the "world's largest" online fitness stores
  - free entry into the 12-week fitness challenge contest
- success stories and testimonials from members and experts
- ACE Diet Plan—nutritional strategies for you designed to promote fat burning processes—customized for age, gender, body-type, personal preferences and schedule, activity level and goals
- get involved and keep current—GHF's *Success Coach* is a motivational service to reduce excuses, fears, procrastination, and emotional baggage that may be holding you back from achieving health and fitness. GHF is updated every day with easy-to-follow fitness tips and articles, recipes, and motivational quotes from famous authors, motivational speakers, and lifetime achievers.

- GHF also features links/information sites for:
  - fitness articles
  - fitness tip of the day
  - recipe of the day
  - motivational quote of the day

9.26 Google.com
http://www.directory.google.com

Google is regarded as one of the world's largest search engines capable of searching "the entire Web". It contains over 30 individual language catalogs of information and searches over in their Web pages.

Once on the google.com Web site, click on "Directory" and then on the "Health" site and go to "Conditions and Diseases" categorized by letter. Click on the letter "o" and then on the topic "obesity" for desired Web pages which may be viewed in "Google page rank order" or in "alphabetical order", or according to "categories" of information on such topics as:

- fat acceptance
- Pickwickian Syndrome
- Prader-Willi Syndrome
- support
- surgery
- treatment services
- weight loss products
- weight loss programs
- weight loss support groups

A selection of key links, reports, information provided under "o" obesity include:
- American Society of Bariatric Physicians—specialists in the medical/surgical treatment of obesity—http://www.asbp.org

- NAASO: North American Association for the Study of Obesity—develops, extends, and disseminates knowledge in the field of obesity—http://www.naaso.org
- understanding adult obesity—http://www.niddk.nih.gov
- federal obesity guidelines—http;//www.nhlbi.nih.gov
- Obesity Meds Research News—http://www.obesity-news.com
- obesity: an eating disorder—http://www.anred.com/obese.html
- ABC's of weight loss psychology—http://www.weight-dieting.org
- Obesity Week—news and comprehensive information about prevention, diagnosis, and treatment of obesity—http://www.obesityweek.org
- Obesity-Diet.com—European-based professional Web site dealing with diet and obesity—http:www.obesity-diet.com

Alternatively, using the general Search site and the topic "obesity selected links, reports, information include:
- help for obesity—convenient and personalized health and diet planning
- understanding adult obesity
- association for morbid obesity support
- obesityhelp.com—obesity resources
- obesity law and advocacy center
- obesity—excess of body fat resulting in an impairment of health
- obesity treatments, diet and nutrition
- complexity of obesity—http://www.interself.com
- obesity news from http://www.obesityweek.org
- ANRED: obesity, is it an eating disorder
- obesity research
- obesity surgery web site
- childhood obesity: causes and prevention
- obesity virus?
- surgery for morbid obesity

- obesity research center—Columbia University
- patient resource: obesity
- childhood obesity symposium: causes and prevention
- obesity tutorial
- obesity in children and teens
- weight loss programs consisting of obesity surgery
- childhood and adolescent obesity
- Lap Band laproscopic obesity surgery
- obesity reviews
- NHLBI obesity guidelines
- NIH obesity and weight loss support site
- weight control and obesity
- understanding-obesity.com
- Pickwickian Syndrome
- breathing disorders in obesity
- sleep apnea syndrome in obesity—http://www.talkaboutsleep.com

Use the Search site for additional information.

9.27 Great Outdoors Recreation Pages (GORP) http://www.gorp.com

GORP features adventure, travel, hiking, national parks recreation, enjoyable destinations, gear, books, and tours which entail physical activity and expenditure of bodily energy. Increased physical activity/exercise is an essential part of weight management and health and the treatment of overweight and obesity. Various sites and links are provided for information on:
- "destination" site:
  - United States
  - World
  - Parks

- Regional Guides
- Weekenders
- "activities" site:
  - top ten
  - hiking
  - biking
  - skiing
- "interests" site:
  - seasonal picks
  - food
  - jobs
  - family
  - expert advice
- "favorites" site:
  - Pacific crest trail
  - Dallas weekender
  - Travel guide
  - Down East Maine
- "community" site:
  - discussion groups
  - GORP tools
  - park ratings
  - trails
  - clubs
  - events
- GORP vacations sites:
  - Costa Rica multisport
  - Maine coast
  - Cooper Canyon ride
  - sea kayaking in British Columbia
  - hiking in the desert, forests, or mountains of California's High Sierras

- hiking or rafting in Grand Canyon National Park
- outdoor adventures in North Carolina's or Colorado's mountains
- top 40 America's white water adventures

Use Search site for additional information.

9.28   Health.gov/Dietary Guidelines
http://www.health.gov/dietaryguidelines

The 5th edition of *Nutrition and Your Health: Dietary Guidelines for Americans*, a joint publication of the Departments of Health and Human Services and U.S. Department of Agriculture, was released May 2000.

A one page Summary of the Guidelines and complete text of *Nutrients and Your Health: Dietary Guidelines for Americans* is now available on the Health.gov Web site in HTML or PDF versions. Also, *Using the Dietary Guidelines for Americans* is available.

Development of the Dietary Guidelines was coordinated by the Office of Disease Prevention and Health Promotion, HHS, and the Center for Nutrition Policy and Promotion, USDA.

Principles of the Dietary Guidelines include links/information on:
- aim for fitness
- aim for a healthy weight
- be physically active each day
- build a healthy base
- let the Pyramid guide your food choices
- choose a variety of grains daily, especially whole grains
- choose a variety of fruits and vegetables daily

- keep food safe to eat
- choose sensibly
- choose a diet low in saturated fat and cholesterol and moderate in total fat
- choose beverages and foods to moderate your intake of sugars/carbohydrates
- choose and prepare foods with less salt
- if you drink alcoholic beverages, do so in moderation

Selected additional US Government Resources for links/information include:
- HHS's gateway to reliable healthy information, including diet, nutrition, healthy lifestyle, and physical activity—http://www.healthfinder.gov
- USDA's gateway to nutrition information—http://www.nutrition.gov
- FDA's gateway to federal food safety information—http://www.foodsafety.gov
- National Cancer Institute—http://www.cancer.gov
- Centers for Disease Control and Prevention—http://www.cdc.gov
- Center for Nutrition Policy and Promotion—http://www.usda.gov/cnpp
- Food and Nutrition Information Center—http://www.nalusda.gov /fnic
- National Heart, Lung, and Blood Institute—http://www.nhlbi.nih.gov

9.29   Health.gov/Healthy People 2010
http://www.health.gov/healthypeople

Healthy People 2010 is a comprehensive set of national health objectives for Americans. This program identifies steps that can be taken to maintain or improve health for ourselves, our families, and our communities. Included are 10 leading health indicators (LHIs). These LHIs are 10 major health issues that represent our greatest public health and individual challenges.

The top 2 LHIs are regarded as :
1. physical activity
2. overweight and obesity

Increased physical activity and reduction in overweight and obesity are specific steps that can be taken for all those concerned for better health and a longer and more enjoyable life. For additional information on LHIs, consult:
http://www.healthfinder.gov

Regarding "physical activity", the leading LHI, consult:
*   President's Council on Physical Fitness and Sports
    http://www.fitness.gov
*   Centers for Disease Control and Prevention (CDC)
    http://www.cdc.gov/nccdphp/dnpa

For "overweight and obesity", consult:
*   Obesity Education Initiative, National Heart, Lung and Blood Institute (NHLBI)
    http://www.nhlbi.nih.gov/about/oei/index.htm
*   Weight-Control Information Network
    http://www.niddk.nih.gov/health/nutrit/win.htm

For additional information, consult:
http://www.health.gov/healthypeople/LHI/lhiwhat.htm

Google.com also provides information on each of the LHIs, searched separately.

9.30   Health on the Net Foundation (HON)
http://www.hon.ch

Health on the Net dates back to September 1995 when 60 renowned participants from 11 countries met in Geneva, Switzerland at a conference entitled: *The Use of the Internet and World-Wide Web for Telematics in Healthcare.* These experts voted unanimously to create a permanent body that would promote effective and reliable use of the Internet/Web for healthcare around the world. The HON Web site became operational some 6 months later on March 20, 1996, and rapidly became one of the very first to guide lay users, patients, and medical professionals to reliable sources of healthcare information on the Web.

HON is now regarded as one of the most respected non-profit Web sites for medical information on the Internet/Web. It is a Swiss foundation, operating out of Geneva, Switzerland with generous support of the local Geneva government, the University Hospitals of Geneva, and the Swiss Institute of Bioinformatics. HON's distinguished guiding Council members and Web team hail from several European countries and the USA.

Distinguishing features of this Web site are:
- two widely-used medical search tools, MedHunt and HonSelect
- HON Code of Conduct for the provision of authoritative, trustworthy, Web-based medical information

Information is provided in English, French, German, Spanish or Portuguese.
In addition, HON offers free access to Medline/PubMed and the ability to search these large public compendiums of medical articles.

Using the HONselect Search site and the word (topic) obesity, four results in MeSH terms are provided for information, namely:
- disease, obesity
- disease, obesity in diabetes
- disease, obesity, morbid
- chemicals and drugs, anti-obesity agents

MeSH Broader Terms sites for information include:
- nutritional disorders
- nutritional and metabolic diseases
- signs and symptoms
- body weight
- body constitution
- physical examination
- diagnosis

MeSH Narrow Terms sites for information include:
- obesity, morbid
- Pickwickian Syndrome
- Pradi-Walli Syndrome

Cross-Reference sites include:
- anti-obesity agents
- appetite depressants
- diet, reducing
- lipectomy
- hyperphagia
- body weight
- eating disorders
- weight gain
- skin-fold thickness

Medline's articles for "obesity" pertain chiefly to:
- etiology
- diagnosis
- therapy
- prognosis

Web resources for "obesity" include:
- American Academy of Family Physicians
  http://www.aafp.org
- *Understanding Adult Obesity* report
  http://www.niddlk.nih.gov
- CTF PHC report: *Detection, Prevention, and Treatment of Obesity*
  http://www.ctfphc.org
- Newton Wellesley Obesity Associates
  http://www.nwobese.com
- HON code—*Obesity Meds and Research News*
  http://www.obesity-news.com
- HON code—obesity week
  http://www.obesityweek.org

Medical News on the topic of "obesity" includes information on:
- gut hormone curbs appetite
- natural fat burner found in mouse study
- excess weight in teens linked to ovarian cancer
- rise in body weight linked directly to heart risk
- making schools healthier can cut obesity in children
- US obesity fight needs help from docs
- obesity doubles colon cancer risk in young women
- before you eat, stop and think: are you hungry
- Americans unaware of obesity
- obese show different hunger hormone response
- scientists may have found way to boost metabolism

- experts tighten obesity guidelines for Asians
- future diabetics face high heart attack risk now

Various clinical trials in obesity are offered by Clinicaltrials.gov including:
- obese patients with type 2 diabetes
- safety and efficacy of xenical in children and adolescents with obesity-related disease
- strength training for obesity-related disease
- meditation-based treatment for binge eating disorder
- supplemental calcium in overweight people
- use of the Internet/Web to facilitate weight loss and maintenance

Use Search site for additional information.

9.31 Healthfinder.gov (HFG)
http://www.healthfinder.gov

Healthfinder was developed in 1997 by the U.S. Department of Health and Human Services in conjunction with other federal agencies. It is recognized as a key resource for finding U.S. government health and human services information on the Internet/Web. It has links to carefully selected information and Web sites from over 1,800 health-related organizations

HFG is coordinated by the Office of Disease Prevention and Health Promotion (ODPHP) with participation of a Steering Committee composed of: 1) representatives of the federal agencies (whose information is used), 2) non-federal consumer health information specialists, 3) librarians and 4) others actively engaged in the provision or use of online consumer health information. Significant support also is provided by the National Health Information Center.

Key information sites provided include:
- search
- health library—health information A to Z
- directory—carefully selected health information Web sites

Click on "health library" and then on the letter "o" and go to "obesity".
Links to information provided include:
- aim for a healthy weight: information for health professionals and patients (NHLBI)
- behavioral risk factors (CDC)
- body fat lab—interactive site where you can learn more about your percent body fat and the role it plays in your overall health, and calculate your body mass index (Shape Up America)
- calculate your body mass index (NHLBI)
- cardiovascular information for patients and the general public (NHLBI)
- choosing a safe and successful weight-loss-program (NIDDK)
- clinical guidelines on the identification, evaluation and treatment of overweight and obesity in adults (NHLBI)
- do you know the risks of being overweight (NIDDK)
- easy-to-read English/Spanish booklets on heart health (NHLBI)
- facts about heart disease and women: reducing high blood cholesterol (NHLBI)
- FDA approves orlistat for obesity (FDA)
- find a bariatric physician (American Society of Bariatric Physicians)
- improving cardiovascular health in African Americans
- information about losing weight and maintaining a health weight (CFSAN)
- information for people 20-64 years old (CFSAN)
- interactive menu planner (NHLBI)
- obesity education initiative: guide to behavioral change (NHBLI)

- prescription medications for the treatment of obesity (NIDDK)
- Surgeon General's call to action to prevent and decrease overweight and obesity (USDHHS)
- watch your weight (NHLBI)
- ways to win at weight loss (FDA)
- weight loss and control (WIN)
- what is your body fat IQ (Shape Up America)

Use Search site for additional information.

9.32 IntelliHealth
http://www.intellihealth.com

Aetna IntelliHealth features Harvard Medical School Consumer Health Information.

Sites featured include:
- search—topics of interest
- diseases and conditions—alphabetical list
- healthy lifestyle—fitness, nutrition, weight management
- your health—children, teens, men's, women's senior's
- look it up—symptoms, medical dictionary, health A-Z, drug resources

Searching the topic "obesity", links/information include:
- what causes obesity
- obesity, basic and complications
- weight management
- sleep apnea
- obesity and heart failure
- obesity, definition
- obesity and depression

- lose pounds to lower risk of complications
- obesity, a national health problem
- prescription medications for treatment of obesity
- gastric surgery for severe obesity
- obesity in American children
- obesity cited in fast food law suit
- weight cycling
- sample menus/various cuisines
- pyramids-a-plenty
- nutrition and obesity
- daily food guide
- heredity and obesity
- health associations and resources and obesity
- dieting and gallstones
- risk factors for diabetes
- nutrition and diet
- meridia for treatment of obesity
- Massachusetts adults becoming more fat
- risk of being overweight
- ephedra in obesity
- senators introduce obesity bill
- school program reduces risk of obesity
- body fat distribution, weight gain and breast cancer survival
- type 2 diabetes and obesity
- strategies to prevent heart disease in obese women
- dietary fat
- exercise
- binge-eating disorders
- coronary artery disease and obesity
- atherosclerosis and obesity
- weight and diet and arthritis
- guide to behavior change in obesity

Use the Search site for additional information.

9.33 Just Move.org (JMO)
http://www.justmove.org

This site contains key information on overweight, obesity, and health-related complications provided by the American Heart Association.

Featured key links/information sites include:
- my fitness
    - low active—for people who don't exercise on a regular basis
    - active—for those who work out 2-3 times a week and enjoy physical activity/exercise
    - special case—things one needs to know to stay healthy
- fitness resources
    - lifestyle/fitness type
    - recommendations for physical activity
    - frequently asked questions and answers
    - health facts
- exercise diary
    - my diary—your exercise progress online
- events
    - American Heart Walk

Searching the topic "obesity", links/information sites include:
- obesity and overweight
- obesity and overweight in children
- fitness news archives
- fitness news: US Surgeon General: obesity at epidemic levels
- fitness news: study ties girl's body weight to early puberty
- fitness news: obesity linked to poor lung function in men
- body composition tests

- risk factors and coronary heart disease
- exercise (physical activity)
- exercise and your heart
- risk factors (statistics on physical inactivity and obesity)
- fitness news: health facts
- exercise in children
- exercise for older people and those with disabilities
- fitness news: sidewalks, parks could boost US exercise rates
- aspirin in heart attack and stroke prevention
- physical activity and cardiovascular health: questions and answers
- AHA scientific position: cholesterol
- benefits of daily physical activity
- just move
- children and physical activity fact sheet
- walking for a healthy heart
- fitness news: exercise helps osteoarthritics stay active
- fitness news: mutant mice "pig out", stay skinny
- fitness news archive

Just Move recommends that you consult with your doctor/health professional to determine what's best for you before engaging in any physical activity/exercise program.

9.34 Karolinska Institute (KI)
http://www.mic.ki.se

Karolinska Institute is Sweden's only university for medicine. It accounts for around 40 per cent of all the medical research at universities throughout Sweden. The KI library is Sweden's largest medical library.

A Search site is provided for MeSH classified resources on the Internet/Web for the general public and healthcare professionals. MeSH –Medical Subject headings—is the US National Library of Medicine's (NLM) controlled vocabulary used to index and catalogue bibliographic and other types of biomedical information. You may use the 2002 MeSH at NLM for overweight, obesity, and health-related complications information to accomplish your search for desired information.

Click on the "alphabetical list of specific diseases/disorders" option, click on the letter "o" and then on the topic "obesity" for links/information including:

- what is obesity
- identification, evaluation, and treatment of overweight and obesity in adults
- information on nutrition and obesity
- clinical guidelines: obesity in adults
- gastroplasty for severe obesity
- North American Association for the Study of Obesity
- Low-carbohydrate diets: heresy or hype
- Xenical (orlistat)
- position statement on obesity
- childhood "globesity"
- evaluation and treatment of childhood obesity
- obesity gene map menu
- neurophysiology of appetite
- control of appetite and eating behavior
- Olwen's links on obesity surgery
- laproscopic gastric Alvarado C bypass surgery for weight control
- obesity surgery: Roux-en-Y gastric bypass procedure
- surgery options for obesity

Those looking for information/guidance are strongly advised to discuss this Web information with their professional physician/healthcare provider.

Use Search site for additional information.

9.35 Librarians' Index to the Internet (LII)
http://www.lii.org

LII is a searchable annotated subject directory of more than 10,000 Internet/Web resources evaluated by librarians for their usefulness and reliability. Since, October 2000, operational funding has been provided by the Library of California and hosting continues to be provided by the University of California at Berkley Sun SITE.

The "Health and Medicine: Diseases and Conditions" site provides links/information on various topics such as "weight loss", "obesity", etc. Clicking on "weight loss", for example, provides links/information on:
*   DietWorldOnline.com (http://www.dietworldonline.com)—diet and weight loss/fitness, etc.—collection of information on losing weight by someone who has been there.
*   TOPS (Take Off Pounds Sensibly) (http://www.tops.org)—an international non-profit weight loss support group in existence since 1948 which does not sell or support any particular products.
*   You Can Control Your Weight as You Quit Smoking—answers to commonly asked questions. Topics discussed include causes of weight gain after quitting, health risks of smoking, benefits of quitting, methods for avoiding weight gain, and ways to reduce cravings for both cigarettes and food. Includes other recommended Web resources for additional information.

Clicking on "obesity" provides links and information on:

- American Obesity Association (http://www.obesity.org)—organization for advocacy, education, and monitoring federal agencies for changes in laws affecting the lives of persons with obesity. Provides information on IRS Ruling 2002-19—obesity is now accepted as a disease and expenses incurred for the diagnosis and treatment may qualify as expenses for medical care subject to the limitations of the ruling.
- American Society of Bariatric Physicians (http://www.asbp.org)—bariatrics view of obesity and its treatment.

Use Search site for additional information.

9.36   Medline (M)
http://medline.cos.com

Medline, compiled by the National Library of Medicine is the world's most comprehensive sources of life sciences and biomedical bibliographic information. It is reported to contain around 11 million records from over 7,300 different publications from 1965 to today. Medline is updated weekly.

Medline through COS (Community of Science) provides links/information on:

- search interfaces for all experience levels
- search or browse Medical Subject Headings (MeSH)
- search by specific medical journals
- download search results in a variety of formats
- Medline abstracts to information in other biological databases
- access COS Query Track which allows you to save your searches from each session and quickly repeat them in future sessions
- obtain abstracts or full published articles on topics of interest

Other links/information sites provided include:
- instructions
- subscribe
- log in for individual subscribers
- help desk
- query track
- Medline fact sheet
- main search
- simple search
- advanced search
- search—specific journals
- browse or search Medline

Medline also may be accessed via the National Library of Medicine (http://www.nlm.nih.gov) or, through Health on the Net Foundation (http://www.hon.ch).

Use the Search site to obtain information on overweight, obesity and health-related topics of interest.

9.37 Medlineplus (MP)
   http://www.nlm.nih.gov/medlineplus

MP is a service of the National Library of Medicine (the world's largest medical library) and National Institutes of Health (a trusted source of medical information), from their online databases involving over 11 million documents. Medlineplus does not accept any advertising on their site nor do they endorse any company or product.

Key links/information sites include:
- dictionaries—provide spellings and definitions of medical terms— also encyclopedias/glossaries

- directories—locations and credentials of doctors
- drug information—generic and brand name drugs used to treat overweight and obesity, and related complications such as type 2 diabetes, hypertension, heart disease, stroke, etc.
- health topics—conditions such as overweight and obesity plus a medical encyclopedia
- other resources—access to organizations, consumer health libraries, international sites, publications, Medline, and more

Dictionaries/encyclopedias/glossaries/links include:
- ADAM Medical Encyclopedia
- Cancer.gov Dictionary (National Cancer Institute)
- Heart and Stroke Encyclopedia (American Heart Association)
- Meriam-Webster Medical Dictionary (Intellihealth)
- Multilingual Glossary of Technical and Popular Medical Terms in Eight European Languages (European Commission)
- On-line Medical Dictionary (Cancer WEB)
- Talking Glossary of Genetic Terms (National Human Genome Research Institute)
- Terms and Definitions (NIH Office of Rare Diseases)
- Word: A Glossary of Medical Words (Nemours Foundation)
- Medical Dictionaries and Glossaries (Jim Martindale)
- Michigan eLibrary—Health and Medical Dictionaries (Michigan Electronic Library)
- Patient Education: Glossaries (DMOZ Open Directory Project)
- Web of Online Dictionaries (Bucknell University)

Clicking on Health Topics A-Z and then on the letter "o" for "obesity", links/information include:
- news
- from NIH
- general/overview

- clinical trials
- diagnosis/symptoms
- nutrition
- prevention/screening
- research
- specific aspects
- treatment
- dictionaries/glossaries
- directories
- journals/newsletters
- organizations
- statistics
- children
- Spanish language
- primary NIH organization for research on obesity is the National Institute of Diabetes and Digestive and Kidney Diseases (NIDDK)
- search Medline for recent research articles on obesity
- obesity
- weight loss/obesity
- food, nutrition, and metabolism

Latest News presents links/reports/information on:
- natural fat burner found in mouse study
- excess weight in teens linked to ovarian cancer
- rise in body weight linked directly to heart risk
- heart study finds strong link between obesity and heart failure (NHLBI)
- drug targets brain circuits that drive appetite and body weight
- high-fat, low-carbohydrate weight loss diet (AHA)
- more news on obesity

From the National Institutes of Health, reports include:
* *Aim for a Healthy Weight: Key Recommendations*
* *Do You Know the Health Risks of Being Overweight*
* *Understanding Adult Obesity*

General/Overviews reports include:
* *Basics About Overweight and Obesity* (from CDC)
* JAMA Patient Page: *Are You Obese* (AMA)
* *Obesity and Overweight: Frequently Asked Questions* (NCCDPHP)

Clinical trials on:
* Clinicaltrials.gov: obesity (NIH)

Diagnosis reports include:
* *Body Mass Index Chart* (NHLBI)
* *Calculate Your Body Mass Index* (NHLBI)

Nutrition reports include:
* *Eating Healthy Starts with Healthy Food Shopping* (NHLBI)
* *Eating Healthy with Ethnic Food* (NHLBI)
* *Weight Control: Eating Right and Keeping Fit* (ACOG)

Preventing/Screening report on:
* *Physical Activity, Good Nutrition and Obesity* (CDC)

Research reports on:
* *Designer Mice Eat More, Weigh Less* (NIGMS)
* *Development of Obesity in Young US Adults* (ACP)
* *Drug Targets Brain Circuits that Drive Appetite and Body Weight* (NIMH)
* *Holiday Weight Gain Slight, but May Last a Lifetime* (NIDDK)

- *Obese Youth have a Condition that Precedes Type 2 Diabetes Mellitus* (NICHHD)
- *Obesity and Heart Failure*—NHLBI Framingham Heart Study
- *Pathological Obesity and Drug Addiction Share Common Brain Characteristics (NIDA)*
- *Trunk Fat Causes Heavy Load for Boys* (AHA)

Specific Conditions/Aspects reports include:
- *Active at Any Size* (WIN)
- *Losing Weight: More than Counting Calories* (FDA)
- *Obesity and Cancer* (NCI)
- *Obesity and Genetics: What We Know, What We Don't Know, and What It Means* (NCEH)
- *Overweight, Obesity Threaten US Health Gains* (FDA)

Treatment reports include:
- *Bariatric Surgery for Morbid Obesity* (AEG)
- *Gastric Surgery for Severe Obesity* (WIN)
- *Implanted Stomach Band to Treat Severe Obesity* (FDA)
- *Prescription Medications for the Treatment of Obesity* (CDER)
- *Very Low-Calorie Diets* (WIN)

Glossary includes:
- *Obesity, Physical Activity and Weight-Control Glossary* (WIN)

Directory includes:
- *Find a Dietician* (ADA)

Print Publication report include:
- *Weight Control and Obesity* (USDA)

Organizations include:
- American Obesity Association (AOA)
- National Heart, Lung and Blood Institute (NHLBI)
- National Institute of Diabetes and Digestive and Kidney Disease (NIDDK)
- Weight-control Information Network (NIDDK)

Statistics reports include:
- FASTATS—*Overweight Prevalence* (NIH)
- *Obesity Continues to Climb in 1999 Among American Adults* (NCCDPHP)
- *Obesity Trends: Prevalence of Obesity* (NIDDK)
- *Diabetes and Obesity Continue to Threaten the Health of Americans* (CDC)

Children reports include:
- *Body Mass Index (BMI) Charts* (Nemours Foundation)
- *Childhood Obesity: Parenting Advice* (Mayo Clinic)
- *Is Your Child Overweight* (AAP)

Use Search site for additional information.

9.38   Mental Help Net (MHN)
   http://www.mentalhelp.net

MHN participates in the Center Site Network of behavioral healthcare websites and from which it receives content. This Web resource is reported to have won a number of awards for excellence.

Featured links/information sites include:
- anxiety disorders
- bipolar disorder

- depression
- eating disorders
- life problems
- mental/psychological disorders
- schizophrenia

Anxiety and/or depression frequently complicate overweight and obesity. Whether or not either or both are the "cause" and/or the "result" remains to be determined in each individual case. Weight gain may also be a side effect of medications used to treat anxiety, depression or other mental disorders. Drugs used to treat bipolar and psychotic disorders frequently cause significant weight gain and even obesity.

Searching the topic "obesity" links/information provided include:
- obesity
- vicious cycle of obesity
- theories about the causes of depression
- references and methods for specific disorders
- when to seek professional help
- psychological self-help
- behavioral medicine treatment planner
- obese children at increased risk for low self-esteem

Use the Search site for additional information.

9.39 National Center for Complementary and Alternative Medicine (NCCAM)
http://www.nccam.nih.gov

NCCAM is one of 27 institutes and centers of the National Institutes of Health (NIH), 1 of 8 agencies under the Public Health Service (PHS) in the Department of Health and Human Services (DHHS). Their mission is to support rigorous research on complementary and alternative medicine (CAM), to train researchers in CAM and to disseminate information to the public and professionals on which CAM modalities, treatments, preventatives work, which do not and why.

Sites featured for links/information include:
- health information
- research
- clinical trials
- news and events
- understanding CAM
- alerts and advisories
- treatment information
- more resources
- clinical trials
- understanding clinical trials
- finding NCCAM clinical trials
- news and events
- press releases
- NCCAM newsletter

Recent reports of interest include
- *Chelation Therapy for Coronary Heart Disease*
- *Ephedra in Dietary Supplements*
- *Consumer Advisory*
- *HHS Plans to Study Ephedra*

Use the Search for additional information.

9.40 National Center on Sleep Disorders Research (NCSDR)
http://www.nhlbi.nih.gov/about/ncsdr

NCSDR is located within the National Heart, Lung, and Blood Institute (NHLBI) of the National Institutes of Health (NIH). It was established in 1993 to help combat a serious public health concern about the growing problem of sleep disorders in America estimated to add billions of dollars annually to the national health bill.

Key sites for links/information include:
*   research
*   professional education
*   patient and public information
*   communications
*   news and press releases
*   clinical guidelines
*   studies seeking patients

The principal sleep disorders complicating obesity links/information are:
*   sleep apnea
*   Pickwickian Syndrome

Other sleep links/information sites of interest include:
*   awake at the wheel
*   facts about problem sleepiness
*   facts about sleep apnea
*   test your sleep IQ
*   sleep apnea video

Further information on sleep apnea or the Pickwickian Syndrome may be obtained from Medlineplus at: http://www.nlm.nih.gov/medlineplus by searching these topics.

The *Facts About Sleep Apnea* report provides an overview regarding: 1) What is sleep apnea?, 2) Who gets it?, 3) What causes it?, 4) Effects, 5) Diagnosis, and 6) Treatment. The report is available at: http://www.nhbli.nih.gov/health/public/sleep/sleepapnea.txt.

The NHLBI report on *Breathing Disorders During Sleep* including information on sleep apnea, its importance, diagnosis, complications, and treatment, is available at: http://www.medhelp.org/lib/breadiso.htm.

9.41   National Guideline Clearinghouse (NGC) http://www.guideline.gov

NGC is a public resource for evidence-based clinical practice guidelines sponsored by the Agency for Healthcare Research and Quality (formerly the Agency for Health Care Policy and Research (AHCPR), in partnership with the American Medical Association (AMA) and the American Association of Health Plans (AAHP).

The NGC provides physicians, nurses, and other health professionals, health care providers, health plans, integrated delivery systems, and others an accessible mechanism for obtaining objective, detailed information on clinical practice guidelines.

Search results for the topic "obesity" provides guidelines by:
- American Association of Clinical Endocrinologists (AACE)/American College of Endocrinology 1997, revised 1998, 35 pages
- *Clinical Guidelines on the Identification, Evaluation and Treatment of Overweight and Obesity in Adults*, NHLBI/NIDDK, 1998, 28 pages

- *Lipoplasty*, American Society of Plastic Surgeons, 1998, 9 *pages*
- *Guidelines for Adolescent Preventive Service (GAPS)*, American Medical Association, 1997, 8 pages
- *Prevention of Coronary Heart Disease in Clinical Practice*, European Society of Cardiology/European Atherosclerosis Society/European Society of Hypertension/European Society of General Practice/Family Medicine/International Society of Behavioral Medicine/European Heart Network, 1998, 70 pages
- *Preventive Counseling and Education*, Institute for Clinical Systems Improvement, 1995, revised 2001, 61 pages
- *Management of Stable Angina: A National Guideline*, Scottish Intercollegiate Guidelines network, 2001, 26 pages
- *Evidence-based Protocol: Exercise Promotion: Walking in Elders*, University of Iowa Gerontological Nursing Interventions Research Center, Research Dissemination Core, 2001, 53 pages
- *Cardiac Rehabilitation*, Agency for Healthcare Research and Quality, 1995, revised 2000, 202 pages
- *Guidelines of Care for Liposuction*, American Academy of Dermatology, 2001, 10 pages
- *Benefits and Risks of Controlling Blood Glucose Levels in Patients with Type 2 Diabetes Mellitus*, American Academy of Family Physicians/ American Diabetes Association, 1999, 39 pages
- *Prevention of Obesity in Adults*, Canadian Task Force on Preventive Health Care, 1999, 12 pages
- *Guidelines for the Clinical Application of Laparoscopic Biliary Tract Surgery*, Society of American Gastrointestinal Endoscopic Surgeons, 1999, 3 pages
- *Third Report of the National Cholesterol Education Program (NCEP), Expert Panel on Detection, Evaluation, and Treatment of High Blood Cholesterol*, NHLBI, 1993, updated 2001.

- *Nutrition Recommendations and Principles for People with Diabetes Mellitus,* American Diabetes Association, 1986, revised 1998, republished 2001, 5 pages
- *Evidence-based Nutrition Principles and Recommendations for the Treatment and Prevention of Diabetes and Related Complications,* American Diabetes Association, 2001, republished 2002, 11 pages

Use Search site for additional information.

9.42 National Heart, Lung and Blood Institute (NHLBI) http://www.nhlbi.nih.gov

The NHLBI provides leadership for national programs regarding heart, blood vessels, blood and blood resources, and sleep disorders. Since 1997, the NHLBI also has had administrative responsibility for the NIH Women's Health Initiative. It plans, conducts, fosters, and supports an integrated and coordinated program of basic research, clinical investigations and trials, observational studies, and demonstration and education projects. Research is dedicated to the causes, prevention, diagnosis, and treatment of heart, blood vessel, lung, blood diseases and sleep disorders.

Links/information sites featured include:
- what's new
- site index
- health information
- scientific resources
- news and press releases
- clinical guidelines
- studies seeking patients
- labs at NHLBI

Click on "Clinical Guidelines" and then *Clinical Guidelines on Overweight and Obesity,* for a full report on the subject. This report also can be found at: http://www.nhlbi.nih.gov/guidelines/obesity/ob_home.htm

Searching the topic "obesity", links and reports include:
* *Calculate Your Body Mass Index (BMI)*
  http://www.nhlbisupport.com/bmi/bmicalc.htm
* *Body Mass Index Table*
  http://www.nhlbi.nih.gov/guidelines/obesity/bmi_tbl2.htm
* *Clinical Guidelines on the Identification, Evaluation, and Treatment of Overweight and Obesity in Adults*
  http://www.nhlbi.nih.gov/guidleines/obesity/ob_home.htm
* *Selecting a Weight Loss Program*
  http://www.nhlbi.nih.gov/health/public/heart/obesity/lose_wt/wtl_prog.htm
* *Aim for a Healthy Weight: Key Recommendations*
  http://www.nhlbi.nih.gov/health/public/heart/obesity/lose_wt/recommen.htm
* *Aim for a Health Weight: Assessing Your Risk*
  http://www.nhlbi.nih.gov/halth/public/heart/obesity/lose_wt/risk.htm
* *Aim for a Health Weight: Controlling Your Weight*
  http://www.nhlbi.nih.gov/health/public/heart/obesity/lose_wt/control.htm
* *Guide to Physical Activity*
  http://www.nhlbi.nih.gov/health/public/heart/obesity/lose_wt/phy_act.htm
* *Aim for a Healthy Weight: Information for Health Professionals*
  http://www.nhlbi.nih.gov/health/public/heart/obesity/lose_wt/profmats.htm

- *Guide to Behavior Changes*
  http://www.nhlbi.nih.gov/health/public/heart/obesity/lose_wt/behavior.htm
- *Shopping: What to Look for*
  http://www.nhlbi.nih.gov/health/public/heart/obesity/lose_wt/shopping.htm
- *Tip Sheets: Eating Healthy (Dining Out, Ethnic Food, Fat and Calories, Healthy Food Shopping)*
  http://www.nhlbi.nih.gov/health/public/heart/obesity/lose_wt/ob_tips.htm
- *Guidelines on Overweight and Obesity: Rationale*
  http://www.nhlbi.nih.gov/guidelines/obesity/e_txtbk/ratnl/20.htm
- *Guidelines on Overweight and Obesity: Treatment Guidelines*
  http://www.nhlbi.nih.gov/guidelines/obesity/e_txtbk/txgd/40.htm
- *Guidelines on Overweight and Obesity: Health and Economic Costs*
  http://www.nhlbi.nih.gov/guidelines/obesity/e_txtbk/ratnl/21.htm
- *Guidelines on Overweight and Obesity: Health Risks of Overweight and Obesity*
  http://www.nhlbi.nih.gov/guidelines/obesity/e_txtbk/ratnl/22.htm
- *Guidelines on Overweight and Obesity: Prevention of Overweight and Obesity*
  http://www.nhlbi.nih.gov/guidelines/obesity/e_txtbk/ratnl/23.htm
- *Guidelines on Overweight and Obesity: Environment*
  http://www.nhlbi.nih.gov/guidelines/obesity/e_txtbk/ratnl/24.htm
- *Guidelines on Overweight and Obesity: Genetic Influence in Development of Overweight and Obesity*
  http://www.nhlbi.nih.gov/guidelines/obesity/e_txtbk/ratnl/25.htm
- *Guidelines on Overweight and Obesity: Management of Weight Loss*
  http://www.nhlbi.nih.gov/guidelines/obesity/e_txtbk/txgd/43.htm
- *Guidelines on Overweight and Obesity: Economic Costs of Overweight and Obesity*
  http://www.nhlbi.nih.gov/guidelines/obesity/e_txtbk/ratnl/213.htm

- *Guidelines on Overweight and Obesity: Goals of Weight Loss and Management*
  http://www.nhlbi.nih.gov/guidelines/obesity/e_txtbk/txgd/431.htm
- *Guidelines on Overweight and Obesity: Strategies for Weight Loss*
  http://www.nhlbi.nih.gov/guidelines/obesity/e_txtbk/txgd/432.htm
- *Guidelines on Overweight and Obesity: Weight Reduction after Age 65*
  http://www.nhlbi.nih.gov/guidelines/obesity/e_txtbk/txgd/452.htm
- *Guidelines on Overweight and Obesity: Smoking Cessation in the Overweight or Obese Patient*
  http://www.nhlbi.nih.gov/guidelines/obesity/e_txtbk/txgd/453.htm
- *Guidelines on Overweight and Obesity: Appendix IV. Obesity and Sleep Apnea*
  http://www.nhlbi.nih.gov/guidelines/obesity/e_txtbk/appndx/apn dx4.htm
- *Guidelines on Overweight and Obesity: Dietary Therapy*
  http://www.nhlbi.nih.gov/guidelines/obesity/e_txtbk/txgd/4321.htm
- *Guidelines on Overweight and Obesity: Physical Activity*
  http://www.nhlbi.nih.gov/guidelines/obesity/e_txtbk/txgd/4322.htm
- *Guidelines on Overweight and Obesity: Behavior therapy*
  http://www.nhlbi.nih.gov/guidelines/obesity/e_txtbk/txgd/4323.htm
- *Guidelines on Overweight and Obesity: Combined Therapy*
  http://www.nhlbi.nih.gov/guidelines/obesity/e_txtbk/txgd4324.htm
- *Guidelines on Overweight and Obesity: Pharmacotheraphy (Drugs)*
  http://www.nhlbi.nih.gov/guidelines/obesity/e_txtbk/txgd/4325.htm
- *Guidelines on Overweight and Obesity: Surgery for Weight Loss*
  http://www.nhlbi.nih.gov/guidelines/obesity/e_ttxbk/txgd/4326.htm

Use the NHLBI's Search site to obtain additional information.

9.43 National Institute on Aging (NIA)
http://www.nia.nih.gov

NIA, founded in 1974, leads a broad scientific effort to understand the nature of aging and to extend the healthy, active years of life. Subsequent amendments to the legislative authority of the NIA designated it as the primary federal agency on Alzheimer's disease research. Alzheimer's disease now is another recognized complication of obesity.

NIA's key mission, among others, is to improve the health and well-being of older Americans through research, and specifically to:
- support and conduct high quality research on:
  - aging process
  - age-related diseases
  - special problems and needs of the aged
- develop and maintain state-of-the art resources to accelerate research progress
- information sites include:
  - health information
  - research programs
  - National Advisory Council on Aging

Searching the topic "obesity" provides a key report on *In Search of the Secrets of Aging* which outlines the relationships of food, oxygen radicals, anti-oxidants and aging, glucose cross linking in tissue, DNA damage/repair, and other factors that may be involved in the aging process and Alzheimer's Disease. This report is available at: http://www.nia.nih.gov/health/pubs/secrets-of-aging/p3.htm.

Other links/information made available via searching "obesity" include:
- women's health and aging
- dealing with diabetes

- what can exercise do for me
- portfolio for progress: reducing disease and disability

Use the Search site to obtain additional information.

9.44   National Institute of Arthritis and Musculoskeletal and Skin Diseases (NIAMS) http://www.niams.nih.gov

NIAMS's mission is to support research into the cause, treatment and prevention of arthritis and musculoskeletal and skin diseases, and the dissemination of information on research progress in these diseases. Osteoarthritis (degenerative arthritis) is a recognized complication of obesity.

Featured links/information sites include:
- Health information—health topics A-Z
- Coalition members
- Research and training
- News and events—highlights, press releases, osteoarthritis initiatives, etc

The Health Topic A-Z site provides links/information on:
- arthritis and diet
- new arthritis drugs for rheumatoid and osteoarthritis
- handout on health: osteoarthritis
- hip replacement
- knee problems
- low back pain
- neck and cervical spine disorder
- now you have a diagnosis: what's next

Use Search site for additional information.

9.45 National Institute of Diabetes and Digestive and Kidney Diseases (NIDDK) http://www.niddk.nih.gov

NIDDK is the NIH steward for medical and behavioral research to extend life and reduce the burdens of illness and disability from diabetes and kidney disease which are recognized major complications of obesity.

Key links/information sites include:

- health information—diabetes, kidney, nutrition, weight loss and control, statistics, etc.—English and Spanish language versions
- National Education Programs—diabetes and kidney disease
- National Information Clearinghouse—diabetes, kidney disease, weight control
- clinical trials—clinicaltrials.gov
- what's new—phenotyping for mouse models of diabetes, diabetic complications, obesity and related disorders
- *Diabetes Prevention Program (DPP)*
- *Health People 2010*

Searching the topic "obesity" provides other reports/information including:
- *Environmental Approaches to the Prevention of Obesity* http://www.niddk.nih.gov/fund/crfo/may2002council/Environme ntal–Approaches–Prevention–Obesity--RFA.htm
- *Obesity Task Force* http://www.niddk.nih.gov/fund/divisions/DDN/obesitytaskforce.htm
- *Boston Obesity/Nutrition Research Center* http://www.niddk.nih.gov/fund/other/centers/boston.*htm*

- *Minnesota Obesity/Nutrition Research Center*
  http://www.niddk.nih.gov/fund/other/centers/minnestoa.htm
- *New York Obesity/Nutrition Research Center*
  http://www.niddk.nih.gov/fund/other/centers/newyork.htm
- *Gastric Surgery for Obesity*
  http://www.niddk.nih.gov/health/nutrit/pubs/gastric/
  gastricsurgergy.htm
- *NIDDK Statistics Related to Overweight and Obesity*
  http://www.niddk.nih.gov/health/nutrit/pubs/statobes.htm
- *Obesity, Physical Activity and Weight-control Glossary*
  http://www.niddk.nih.gov/health/nutrit/pubs/glossary/
  glossaryintro.htm
- *NIDDK Health Information: Weight Loss Control: Long Term
  Studies of Pharmacotherapy for the Management of Obesity*
  http://www.niddk.nih.gov/health/nutrit/table.htm
- *Understanding adult obesity*
  http://www.niddk.nih.gov/health/nutrit/pubs/unders.htm
- *Obesity associated with high rates of diabetes in the Pima Indians*
  http://www.niddk.nih.gov/health/diabetes/pima/obesity/obesity.htm
- *University of Pittsburgh Obesity/Nutrition Research Center*
  http://www.niddk.nih.gov/fund/other/centers/pitt.htm
- *Gastric Surgery for Severe Obesity*
  http://www.niddk.nih.gov/health/nutrit/pubs/gastsurg.htm
- *Prescription Medications for the Treatment of Obesity*
  http://www.niddk.nih.gov/health/nutrit/pubs/presmeds.htm
- *Health Information: Weight Loss and Control*
  http://www.niddk.nih.gov/health/nutrit/nutrit.htm
- *Very Low-calorie Diets*
  http://www.niddk.nih.gov/health/nutrit/pubs/vlcd.htm
- *Walking: A Step in the Right Direction*
  http://www.niddk.nih.gov/health/nutrit/walking/walkingbro/walk
  ing2.html

- *Dieting and Gallstones*
  http://www.niddk.nih.gov/health/nutrit/pubs/dietgall.htm
- *Health Information: National Diabetes Information Clearinghouse*
  http://www.niddk.nih.gov/health/diabetes/ndic.htm
- *Health Information: Diabetes*
  http://www.niddk.nih.gov/health/diabetes/diabetes.htm
- *Risk Factors for Non Insulin-dependent Diabetes*
  http://www.niddk.nih.gov/health/diabetes/dia/chpt9.pdf
- *Do You Know the Health Risks of Being Overweight*
  http://www.niddk.nih.gov/health/nutrit/pubs/health.htm
- *Weight Loss and Control*
  http://www.niddk.nih.gov/health/nutrit/nutrit.htm

Use the Search site for additional information.

9.46   National Institutes of Health (NIH)
http://www.health.nih.gov

NIH comprises 25 Institutes and Centers and is the leading federal research effort concerning medical research in the United States.

Featured links/information sites include:
- health information
- news and events
- Institutes, Centers and Offices

To learn about health conditions, click-on one or more of the following sites and search their databases for information on overweight, obesity and health-related complications of interest:
- Health Information Index—health topics A-Z and the particular institutes or centers that research them

- Consumer Health Publications—free fact sheets, brochures, and handbooks
- Medlineplus—health resource maintained by the Department of Health and Human Services (DHHS)
- NIH Word on Health—articles on health maintenance and prevention

To participate in research studies, click-one or more of the sites provided (e.g. clinicaltrials.gov, etc.)

Click-on "drug information"—which leads to Medlineplus guide to over 9000 medications including those used in the treatment of overweight, obesity and health-related complications.

A key *Consensus Statement 60: Diet and Exercise in Non-Insulin Dependent Diabetes Mellitus* is available at: http://consensus.nih.gov/cons/060/060_statement.htm.

Use Search site for additional information.

9.47   National Institute of Mental Health (NIMH) http://www.nimh.nih.gov

NIMH is the premier federal effort concerned with mental health research and dissemination of information. Its mission is to diminish the burden of mental illness through basic and clinical research. NIMH strives to translate this basic and clinical knowledge gained from research into better understanding and treatment that ultimately will be effective in our complex world with its diverse populations and evolving healthcare system.

Mental disorders are believed to represent four of the ten leading causes of disability for persons age 5 and older. Among developed nations, including the United States, major depression is held to be a leading cause of disability. Also near the top of the rankings are manic-depressive (bipolar), schizophrenia, and obsessive-compulsive disorder. The NIMH conducts extensive research programs in these and other mental disorders.

Anxiety and depression may initiate overweight, obesity and health-related complications and/or even be a complication of these disorders. In addition, significant weight gain, overweight and obesity may be side effects of psychotropic medications given to patients with mental disorders. Appetite suppressants given to patients for the treatment of overweight and obesity may produce significant central nervous system side effects and abuse.

Key links/information sites featured include:
- breaking news
- clinical trials
- research fact sheets
- information on mental disorders

Searching the topic "obesity", on the NIMH Search site provides key links/information on:
- depression and diabetes and heart disease
- appetite suppressants and body weight
- behavior modification in treatment of obesity
- anxiety and/or depression in overweight and obesity
- psychotropic drug treatment of mental disorders and overweight and obesity

Use the Search site for additional information.

9.48 National Institute of Neurological Disorders and Stroke (NINDS)
http://www.ninds.nih.gov

NINDS, created in 1950, conducts and supports research on brain and nervous system disorders.

High blood pressure and stoke are recognized complications of obesity. A stroke occurs when the blood supply to a part of the brain is interrupted (ischemic stroke) or when a blood vessel in the brain bursts, spilling blood into the spaces surrounding the brain cells (hemorrhagic stroke).

Generally there are 3 treatment stages for stroke, namely: 1) prevention, 2) therapy immediately after stroke, and 3) post-stroke rehabilitation. For further information click on the "stroke" site or consult: http://www.ninds.nih.gov/heatlh_and_medicaldisorders/stroke.htm

The "Stroke Information Page" provides links/information on:
- what is stroke
- is there any treatment
- what is the prognosis
- what research is being done
- organizations concerned with various aspects of stroke
- related publications and information.

Related publications includes reports on:
- *Stroke, Hope Through Research*
- *Stroke, Risk Factors and Symptoms*
- *Brain Basics: Preventing Stroke*
- *Transient Ischemic Attack*
- *Multi-Infarct Dementia*

• *Report of Stroke Progress Review Group*

Use the Search site for additional information.

9.49 National Library of Medicine (NLM)
http://www.nlm.nih.gov

NLM is the world's largest medical library and creator of Medline/PubMed and Medlineplus. Featured links/information sites include:
• health information—Medline, PubMed, Medlineplus
• library services—catalog, databases, and network of libraries
• research programs
• news and noteworthy
• general information

Medline/PubMed sites provide access to over 11 million NLM/Medline citations, indexing major medical, biological, and other life sciences journals dating back to the mid-1960s, and links to many other sites providing full text articles and other related resources.

PubMed site provides abstracts to published medical/scientific articles.

Medlineplus site provides summary information and references on overweight, obesity and health-related topics as well as anti-obesity/anorectic drug information.

Clinicaltrials.gov site provides information about clinical research studies in obesity.

Other links/information sites include:

- news—from the NY Times, AP News, Reuters health information and others
- organizations—providing health information
- government—health sites from other nations such as NHS Direct (United Kingdom), Canadian Health Network (Canada) and HealthInsite (Australia).

A separate information link is provided for "health professionals".

Use the Search site for additional information.

9.50 National Women's Health Information Center (NWHIC)
http://www.4women.org

NWHIC is a service of the Office on Women's Health in the Department of Health and Human Services. It provides a gateway to the vast array of federal and other women's health information resources. This site helps you to link, read, and download a wide variety of women's health-related information developed by the Department of Health and Human Services, other federal agencies, and private sector resources. NWHIC serves the entire United States, Puerto Rico and the US Virgin Islands and remains a reliable source for women's health information. Information provided is not intended to be used for diagnosis or treatment of a health problem or as a substitute for consulting a licensed medical professional.

Links/information sites featured include:
- hot topics—physical activity, etc.
- press releases
- dictionaries
- body wise

Searching the topic "obesity", reports include:
* *Binge Eating Disorder: Current Knowledge and Future Directions*
  http://www.niddk.nih.gov/health/nutrit/pubs/binge.htm
* *Calculate Your Body Mass Index*
  http://www.nhlbisupport.com/bmi
* *Clinical Guidelines on the Identification, Evaluation and Treatment of Overweight and Obesity in Adults*
  http://www.nhbli.nih.gov/guidelines/obestiy/ob_home.htm
* *Gastric Surgery for Severe Obesity*
  http://www.niddk.nih.gov/health/nutrit/pubs/gastsurg.htm
* *Long-term Pharmacotherapy in the Management of Obesity*

Use the Search site for additional information.

9.51   PubMed (PM)
http://www.ncbi.nlm.nih.gov/pubmed

PM was developed by the National Center for Biotechnology Information (NCBI) at the National Library of Medicine (NLM), located at the National Institutes of Health (NIH). PubMed was designed to provide access to citations from biomedical literature. Subsequently, a linking feature, LinkOut was added to provide access to full-text articles at journal web sites, and other related web resources. LinkOut is a jumping off point from PubMed citations to relevant resources on the Web, such as, full text articles, library holdings, commentaries, author biographies, practice guidelines, consumer health information, and research tools.

As a service of the National Library of Medicine, PM provides access to over 11 million Medline citations dating back to the mid-1960s and additional life science journals. It includes links to many sites providing full text articles and other related resources. PubMed also provides access to Medline.

While abstracts of articles are provided free of charge, user registration, and a fee may be required to access the full text articles for some journals. Free access to Medline and full text articles may be available through other Web resources such as Health-on-the-Net Foundation at: http://www.hon.ch.

Use the Search site for additional information.

9.52 President's Council on Physical Fitness and Sports (PCPFS)
http://www.fitness.gov

Physical activity and fitness for all is the mission of PCPFS. It serves as a catalyst to promote, encourage, and motivate Americans of all ages to become physically active and fit by:

- emphasizing the importance of physical activity/fitness and exercise and the relationship to good health
- increasing physical activity participation and opportunities by encouraging the development of community, recreation, physical fitness and sports programs
- promoting physical activity and fitness in schools by encouraging innovative health and physical education programs
- stimulating needed research studies in sports medicine, physical activity, fitness, and sports performance
- collaborating with business, industry, government and labor organizations on innovative programs to reduce the financial and health care costs associated with physical inactivity

- cooperating with medical and health care professional associations to encourage patient counseling on sound physical activity and fitness habits and practices

Featured sites for links to reports and other information include:
- *Physical Activity Fundamental to Preventing Disease*
- *Healthy People 2010*
- *Ten Tips to Healthy Eating and Physical Activity*
- *The President's Challenge*
- *HHS Weekly Report*
- *President's Council Fact Sheet*
- *Physical Activity Fact Sheet*
- news releases
- other federal publications on:
  - physical activity
  - fitness
  - health
  - nutrition
  - sports
- *Exercised Lately*—video of a life without physical activity
- *See Why Physical Activity Matters*—resources for coaches, teachers, healthcare fitness professionals and parents
- *Learn About the Active Life*—exercise, physical activity and health information designed to help you feel great
- *Tips for Fit Kids*—easy exercises and nutrition tips to urge the younger crowd to get up and get out

9.53 Recreation.Gov (FG)
http://www.recreation.gov

Features recreational and physical activity opportunities on US Government lands.

FG is a partnership among various agencies aimed at providing a single, easy-to-use Web site with information about public recreation areas. The site allows you to search for recreation areas by state, by recreational activity, by agency or by map

Click-on "recreation search" and "find the perfect spot" for recreation and physical activity for you. Search by state, activity, or agency. "Site of the Week" information is featured. Use the "Quick Search" site for additional information.

9.54   Shape Up America (SUA)
http://www.shapeup.org

Founded in 1994, SUA is a non-profit organization dedicated to promoting healthy weight and increased physical activity for life. It is a broad-based coalition of industry, medical/health, nutrition, physical fitness, and related organizations and experts. Stated objectives are to: 1) promote a new understanding of the health importance of achieving and maintaining a healthy weight and increasing physical activity, 2) inform others of proven ways to achieve a healthy body weight, and 3) increase cooperation among national and community organizations committed to advancing healthy weight and increased physical activity as major health priorities.

Links/information sites featured include:
- diabetes
- fitness center
- frequently asked questions and answers
- media
- members
- professional center

The "Fitness Center" provides information on:
* assessing your readiness for exercise , activity level, flexibility, strength, endurance and aerobic fitness
* overcoming common barriers to physical activity
* designing an improvement program that suits your personal goals and objectives
* assisting you in learning what to eat to maximize your workout
* adding exercise into your daily life

The "diabetes connection" provides information on the link between type 2 (non insulin- dependent) diabetes mellitus and obesity. It is estimated that 85-95% of all cases of type 2 diabetes are attributable to overweight/obesity.

The SUA program teaches how to limit portion sizes, make wiser food choices, and adopt a more physically active lifestyle—all of which can help to promote weight loss, weight maintenance and help better manage type 2 diabetes and other complications.

9.55   Tufts Nutritional Navigator (TNN)
   http://navigator.tufts.edu

TNN is a rating guide for nutritional Web sites. It was developed by the Tufts University Gerald and Dorothy R. Friedman School of Nutritional Science and Policy, which is a respected academic center for nutritional excellence, and is underwritten by a grant from Kraft Foods, Inc.

TNN's rating and review guide allows you to: 1) quickly find nutritional information that is best suited to your needs on the Web, 2) sort through volumes of nutritional information to find the most useful for you, and 3) have confidence and trust in the information you obtain.

Web sites featured on TNN are reviewed by Tufts nutritionists who apply rating and evaluation criteria developed by the Tufts University Nutrition Navigator Advisory Board, a prestigious panel of leading US and Canadian nutrition experts. Information is updated quarterly to ensure ratings take into consideration the changing Web and nutrition environments.

Key links/information sites featured include:
- news
- hot topics
- general nutrition
- family
- women
- men
- journalists
- health professionals
- educators
- special dietary needs

Use the Search site for additional information.

9.56   USDA Center for Nutrition Policy Promotion (CNPP) http://www.usda.gov/cnpp

CNPP was created by the US Department of Agriculture (USDA) in December 1994. It is the focal point within the USDA where scientific research provides nutrition information to the American public and others. CNPP carries out its mission by:
- developing and coordinating nutrition policy with the USDA
- investigating techniques for effective nutrition communication
- evaluating the nutrient content of the US food supply

- preparing periodic updates on the cost of family food plans and raising children
- assessing the cost-effectiveness of government sponsored nutrition programs concerning food consumption, expenditures, behavior and nutritional status

CNPP publishes the *Family Economics and Nutrition Review* and *Dietary Guidelines for Americans.*

Key click on links/reports featured include:
- *ABCs of the Dietary Guidelines 2000*
- *USDA Supports 5 a Day for Better Health*
- *How Much Are You Eating*
- *Dietary Guidelines for Americans 2000, 5th edition*
- *Interactive Healthy Eating Index*
- *Recipes and Tips for Healthy, Thrifty Meals*
- *Nutritional Insights*
- *Dietary Guidelines*
- *Food Guide Pyramid*
- *Food Guide Pyramid—For Young Children*
- *Thrifty Food Plans*
- *Childhood Obesity Proceedings*
- *Breakfast and Learning in Children*
- *Nutrition and Aging*
- *Diet and Gene Interactions*
- *Dietary Behavior: Why We Choose the Foods We Eat*
- "Great Nutrition Debate"—a video

Links to other Web Resources, reports and information also are provided. Use the Search site for additional information.

9.57　USDA Food and Nutrition Information Center (FNIC)
http://www.nal.usda.gov/fnic

The FNIC is located at the National Agriculture Library (NAL), a part of the US Department of Agriculture (USDA) and the Agricultural Research Service (ARS). FNIC is supported in part by a Cooperative Agreement with the University of Maryland's Department of Nutrition and Food Science in the College of Agriculture and Natural Resources. Its mission, since 1971, has been to collect and disseminate information about food and human nutrition. This site is updated daily.

FNIC is a leader in online global nutrition information. It is one of several information centers located at the National Agricultural Library (NAL), Agricultural Research Service (ARS), United States Department of Agriculture (USDA). It includes registered dieticians who provide information on food, human nutrition, and food safety.

FNIC Web site has over 1,800 links to current, reliable nutrition information on:
- what's new
- topics A-Z
- FNIC Resource Lists
- dietary supplements
- food composition
- Dietary Guidelines
- Food Guide Pyramid
- FNIC databases
- consumer corner
- teachers click here
- child care nutrition resource system
- food safety
- WIC Works Resource System

- Healthy School Meals Resource System
- Food Stamp Nutrition Connection
- National Agriculture Library

Use the Search site for additional information.

9.58 USDA Nutrient Data Laboratory (NDL) http://www.nal.usda.gov/fnic/foodcomp

NDL is one of seven units in the Beltsville Human Nutrition Research Center (BHNRC) of the Agricultural Research Service (ARS), involved in compiling and developing food composition databases for over a century, along with its predecessor organizations in USDA. Major project of NDL is to maintain USDA National Nutrient Databank. Also, it seeks to improve the quantity and quality of the nutrient data in the databank in cooperation with the National Heart, Lung and Blood Institute (NHLBI) via the National Food and Nutrient Analysis Program (NFNAP).

Today NDL is a repository of information for 100 nutrients and over 7,300 foods.

Key information sites featured include:
- nutritive value of foods
- USDA food composition publications
- frequently asked questions and answers
- food composition and nutrition resource links
- glossary of terms
- measurement conversions tables
- new key foods paper

Use the Search site for additional information.

9.59   US Department of Health and Human Services (DHHS)
http://www.os.dhhs.gov

DHHS is the United States government's principal agency for protecting the health of all Americans and providing essential human services, especially for those who are least able to help themselves.

Among DHHS Operating Divisions are:
- National Institutes of Health (NIH)
- Food and Drug Administration (FDA)
- Centers for Disease Control and Prevention (CDC)
- Agency for Healthcare Research and Quality (AHRQ)

Searching the topic "obesity", reports available include:
- *Healthy People 2010*
- *Campaign to Increase Physical Activity*
- *Overweight and Obesity Threatens US Health Gains*
- *Community Partnerships to Improve Physical Activity*
- *Initiative to Build Healthy Communities*
- *Benefits of Physical Activity for Disease Prevention*
- *Pediatric Growth Charts to Ward Off Future Weight Problems*
- *CDC's role in combating obesity*
- *Diabetes*
- *HHS Promotes Health Through Physical Activity*

DHHS report on *Physical Activity Fundamental to Preventing Disease* is available at: http://aspe.hhs.gov/health/reports/physicalactivity.

9.60   US Surgeon General's Office (SGO)
http://www.surgeongeneral.gov/sgoffice.htm

The Office of the Surgeon General oversees the 6,000-member Commissioned Corps of the US Public Health Service. It is part of the Office of Public Health and Science, US Department of Health and Human Services.

Links/information sites featured are:
* being healthy
* publications
* news and public affairs
* search special topics

Key click on links/reports include:
* *Overweight and Obesity: The Surgeon General's Initiative*
  http://www.sgobesity.niddk.nih.gov
* *Surgeon General's Healthy Weight Advice for Consumers*
  http://www.surgeongeneral.gov/topics/obesity/calltoaction/ fact_advice.htm
* *Overweight and Obesity: A Vision for the Future*
  http://www.surgeongeneral.gov/topics/obesity/calltoaction/ fact_vision.htm
* *Overweight and Obesity: At a Glance*
  http://www.surgeongeneral.gov/topics/obesity/calltoaction/ fact_glance.htm
* *Overweight and Obesity: Health Consequences*
  http://www.surgeongeneral.gov/topics/obesity/calltoaction/ fact_consequences.htm
* *Overweight and Obesity: What You Can Do*
  http://www.surgeongeneral.gov/topics/obesity/calltoaction/ fact_whatcanyoudo.htm

- *Overweight in Children and Adolescent*
  http://www.surgeongeneral.gov/topics/obesity/calltoaction/
  fact_adolescents.htm

Use the Search site to obtain additional information.

9.61 Vegetarian Resource Group (VRG)
http://www.vrg.org

VRG is a nonprofit organization dedicated to educating the public on vegetarianism and interrelated issues of health, nutrition, ecology, ethics and world hunger. Their health professionals, activists, and educators work with businesses and individuals to bring about healthy changes in the schools, workplace, and community in which you live. Registered dieticians and physicians aid in the development of nutrition related publications and books, and answer media questions about the vegetarian diet. Tufts University Nutrition Center has rated this Web site with their highest possible rating.

Featured links/information sites include:
- frequently asked questions and answers
- vegetarian nutrition
- protein and vitamin B-12 in the vegan diet
- vegetarian recipes
- ingredient information
- teens, family and kids
- vegan general information
- restaurants and travel
- food service
- vegan meals for one or two
- guide to fast food
- guide to food ingredients

- vegan nutrition in pregnancy and childhood
- raising a vegetarian family
- feeding vegan children
- vegetarian nutrition for seniors
- VRG news
- vegetarian journal

Use the Search site to obtain additional information.

9.62   Web MD
http://www.webmd.com

WebMD is a leading provider of online health, research and educational information for physicians and consumers. With more than 15 million visitors every month, WebMD is regarded as a leading commercial consumer-focused healthcare information Web site providing useful healthcare information that may help patients play an active role in managing their own health matters in consultation with their physician/healthcare provider. The WebMD content staff uses board-certified physicians and award-winning journalists to process/provide information.

Featured links/information sites include:
- WebMD Health
- Medscape from WebMD
- Condition Centers
- Health Tools

"Medical, Health and Wellness" links/information sites include:
- diseases and conditions
- medical library
- drugs and herbs

- family genetics
- health guide A-Z
- health tools
- clinical trials
- food and nutrition
- women, men, aging
- sports and fitness
- Dean Ornish, MD Lifestyle

"Disease and Conditions" site features comprehensive information on "obesity" including:
- obesity overview
- healthy weight
- classification
- who is affected
- frequently asked questions and answers
- genetics
  - what is obesity
  - when obesity runs in families
  - what genes are involved
  - environmental factors
    - physical activity
    - energy intake
    - culture
    - fetal programming
- health risks associated with obesity
- fat but still fit
- setting goals for weight loss
- first federal obesity guidelines
- choosing a safe and successful weight-loss program

- lose fat in a flash—here's how
- hypnosis
- the facts on diet fads
- weight loss—without fad diets
- nutrition in a can
- helping yourself with a healthful diet
- protein-sparing diet
- non-prescription diet aids
- making the decision about using medications
- prescription weight loss medicine
- obesity medications
  - sibutramine (meridia) and orlistat (xenical)
  - other prescription appetite suppressants
- surgery
  - overview
  - bariatric surgery
  - stomach stapling (restriction) operations
  - gastric bypass

Use the Search site for additional information.

10. Medical Dictionary, Medical Encyclopedia and Glossary

For a Medical Dictionary, Medical Encyclopedia, or Glossary, regarding definitions of terms used in this book, consult:
- Medlineplus
  http://www.nlm.nih.gov/medlineplus
- National Heart, Lung and Blood Institute: Glossary of Terms
  http://www.nhlbi.nih.gov/guidelines/obesity/e_txtbk/appndx/apndx8.htm
- National Library of Medicine
  http://www.nlm.nih.gov

- National Institute of Diabetes and Digestive and Kidney disease
  http://www.niddk.nih.gov/health/nutrit/pubs/glossary/
  glossaryintro.htm
- Other Web Resources in the Author's List

About the Author

Eugene A. DeFelice, M.D., F.A.P.M., author, educator, Distinguished Clinical Professor of Medicine, Fellow of Academy of Psychosomatic Medicine and Fellow American Geriatric Society, is listed in the Manquis' 1) *Who's Who in Medicine and Healthcare*, 2) *Who's Who in America*, and 3) *Who's Who in the World*. He is the author of numerous medical/scientific publications and 8 key medical books.

0-595-26240-6

www.ingramcontent.com/pod-product-compliance
Lightning Source LLC
Chambersburg PA
CBHW061356280526
45784CB00001B/277